TABLE OF CONTENT

Anatomy of the Eyes

To understand how to properly care for our eyes and address issues like dark circles, puffiness, and wrinkles, we must first understand the anatomy of the eyes. This section will provide an overview of the key structures and functions of the eyes to build a foundation before diving into specific eye care treatments.

The Orbits

The orbits are the bony cavities in the skull that contain and protect the eyeballs and associated muscles, vessels, and nerves. The orbits are composed of seven different bones - the zygomatic bone, maxillary bone, palatine bone, ethmoid bone, lacrimal bone, frontal bone, and sphenoid bone. These bones come together to create the four walls and pyramidal structure that encases each eye.

At the apex of the bony orbit lies the optic canal, which allows the optic nerve to pass from the back of the eye to the brain. The orbits provide both protection for the fragile structures of the eye, as well as anchoring points for the muscles that control eye movement.

Eye Muscles

Six extraocular muscles control the movement of each eyeball. These muscles originate at the back of the orbit and insert into the tough outer layer of the eyeball known as the sclera. The six muscles are:

- Medial rectus - rotates the eye inward (toward the nose)
- Lateral rectus - rotates the eye outward (toward the ear)
- Superior rectus - rotates the eye upward

- Inferior rectus - rotates the eye downward
- Superior oblique - rotates the eye downward and outward
- Inferior oblique - rotates the eye upward and outward

The coordinated action of these muscles allows the eyes to move in precise ways to maintain gaze, track objects, and maintain binocular vision.

The Eyeball

Though small in size, the eyeball houses incredibly intricate and specialized equipment that makes vision possible. The main components include:

Fibrous Tunic

The outermost layer of the eye is the fibrous tunic, composed of the white sclera and clear cornea.

The sclera provides structure and protection for the inner contents of the eye. Tendons of the extraocular muscles insert directly into the sclera, allowing the muscles to move the eyeball.

The cornea is the transparent window on the front surface of the eye that allows light to enter. Its curved shape bends and focuses incoming light.

Vascular Tunic

Underlying the fibrous tunic is the vascular tunic, containing blood vessels that nourish eye tissues. The vessels are contained in the choroid, ciliary body, and iris.

The choroid is a thin, pigmented vascular layer adhered to the sclera. In addition to supplying blood, the choroid contains melanin that absorbs excess light to reduce internal reflection in the eye.

The ciliary body is a ring-like thickening of the choroid near the front of the eye. It contains smooth muscle that controls accommodation for near vision and secretes aqueous humor to nourish eye tissues.

The iris, the colored part of the eye, controls the amount of light entering by adjusting the size of the central opening called the pupil. The intrinsic musculature of the iris causes the pupil to constrict and dilate.

Inner Tunic

The innermost layer is the neural tunic, containing specialized nervous tissue for reception and transmission of visual stimuli. The main components are the retina and the optic nerve.

The retina contains over 120 million rods and cones for light reception, allowing us to see images. The subsequent layers of retinal neurons process and transmit these visual signals to the optic nerve.

The optic nerve carries impulses from the retina back to the brain where they are interpreted as vision. The unique wiring system that links photoreceptors in the retina to nerve cells allows us to see color, light, dark and shapes.

Accessory Structures

In addition to the eyeball and orbit, important accessory structures enable and protect eye function.

Eyelids

The upper and lower eyelids protect the front of the eyes from injury and help spread tears across the surface of the eye for lubrication. The lids have special oil glands along their margins to prevent tears from overflowing.

Blinking helps spread tears, clean debris from the eye surface, and maintain moisture on the exposed cornea. The inner surfaces of the lids contain specialized conjunctival tissue that secretes mucus and tears.

Lacrimal System

The lacrimal system produces tears to lubricate and nourish the eye surface and lids. Tears also contain antibacterial agents and enhance optical properties.

Lacrimal glands above each eye secrete the watery layer of tears. Smaller accessory glands in the conjunctiva add an additional layer. Drainage occurs through tiny puncta on the lids that lead to canaliculi and eventually the nasolacrimal duct.

Extraocular Fat and Fascia

Cushioning orbital fat surrounding the eyeball provides shock absorption and eye stabilization within the bony socket. Connective tissue septa divide the fat into compartments. The fascia lining the orbit controls movement of this fatty cushion.

Eye Conditions

Now that we understand eye anatomy, we can better comprehend common eye conditions like dark circles, puffiness, and wrinkling:

- Dark circles - Caused by blood vessels showing through thin under-eye skin, pooling of blood in orbit, pigment changes, and shadowing from sagging fat pads.
- Puffiness - Results from fluid accumulation due to allergies, sleep deprivation, high salt intake, or laxity in orbital septum allowing fat pads to protrude.
- Wrinkling - Dermal degradation and loss of collagen in the under eye area creates an aged, wrinkled appearance.

With this foundation on eye structures and functions, we can now explore treatments targeting renewal and rejuvenation of the entire eye zone. Understanding the anatomy provides insight on how various solutions can help alleviate dark circles, puffiness, wrinkles and other eye concerns.

Common Eye Issues

Now that we have reviewed eye anatomy, we can better understand some of the most prevalent issues that affect the eye area leading to concerns like dark circles, puffiness, and wrinkled or aging skin. Being aware of common eye problems helps us recognize signs and determine appropriate treatment options.

Allergies

Allergies cause inflammation and irritation in the eyes. Particles like pollen, pet dander, or dust mites trigger antibody release, causing blood vessels in the conjunctiva to dilate and permeability to increase. This allows fluids to accumulate in eye tissues leading to redness, swelling, puffiness, and watery eyes. Allergy symptoms may range from mild itchiness and puffiness to more severe swelling that can cause the upper lids to droop or the lower lids to become pulled down from built up fluid. The rubbing and skin irritation associated with allergies can also contribute to dark circles and wrinkles over time.

Dry Eye Syndrome

Dry eye syndrome, or keratoconjunctivitis sicca, occurs when tear production is inadequate or tear film stability is disrupted. Causes range from inflammation, age-related changes, environmental exposures, and medications. Symptoms include stinging, burning, light sensitivity, distorted vision, and soreness.

If the watery layer of tears is not sufficiently coating the eye surface, it leads to irritation of the corneal surface. In response, the damaged corneal nerves send signals to the lacrimal glands to produce more tears, resulting in reflex tearing. This combination of inadequate hydrating tears with instances of reflex watering is the hallmark of dry eyes.

Over time, the struggle with dry eye creates strain lines at the corners of the eyes and accelerates wrinkling of the thin undereye skin.

Eye Strain

Eye strain, or asthenopia, refers to a group of symptoms related to overuse of the eyes for near work. Symptoms arise from effort to maintain eye positioning, accommodation, convergence, and prolonged use. Common complaints with eye strain include sore eyes, blurred vision, headaches, watery eyes, and irritation of the ocular surface.

Contributing factors include uncorrected refractive error, poor lighting, digital screen overuse, improper workstation setup, and underlying dry eye issues. Often eye strain sufferers instinctually wide open and raise their eyebrows in an attempt to see more clearly. Over years, this compounded facial tension etches lines across the forehead and furrows between the brows.

The squinting and pressure also gradually allow the undereye tissues to descend and accumulate fluid, leading to characteristic changes like sunken eyes, dark circles, eye bags and puffy lids.

Eye Injuries & Trauma

The eyes and surrounding structures are vulnerable to injury and trauma which can have devastating ocular consequences as well as visible damage to the supporting facial tissues. Corneal abrasions, chemical splashes, and blunt force are common mechanisms of direct eye injury and post-traumatic inflammation.

However, injury to the eye region extends beyond the globes themselves. Contusions to the thinner undereye skin easily rupture small vessels, creating vivid bruising and swelling. The socket bones can fracture, disrupt orbital fat pads, and tear connective tissue retaining bands in the eyelids. Violent injury often results in tissue laxity, hollowness, and dark shadows. Additionally, surgery or nerve damage during trauma may cause impaired blinking and lubrication leading to dry spots, keratopathy, and tear film abnormalities - ultimately accelerating aging changes.

Eye Lid Disorders

There are various disorders affecting the eyelids that may contribute to circles, bags, and wrinkling:

- Ptosis - drooping of the upper eyelid, sometimes impairing vision, caused by levator muscle dysfunction, nerve damage, or aging.
- Ectropion - eversion and sagging of the lower lid exposing the inner moist surface. This is attributed to horizontal lower lid laxity.
- Entropion - inversion of the lid margin causing lashes to rub against the eye. This results from orbicularis muscle imbalance and horizontal upper or lower lid laxity.
- Blepharochalasis - stretching and atrophy of the tissue connecting the eyelid to the bone, leading to bagginess.

These disorders allow protrusion or distortion of orbital fat, contribute to lower lid retraction and effacement of the lower sulcus. This makes the undereye area appear hollow, darkened, and wrinkled.

As we can see, a wide variety of common eye conditions contribute to the characteristic signs of aging like dark circles, puffiness, and undereye wrinkling over time through inflammation, trauma, and repetitive strain to the delicate tissues surrounding the eye. Understanding the root causes guides our exploration of treatment options for rejuvenation.

Causes of Circles, Puffiness & Wrinkles

Now that we have a solid foundation in eye anatomy and common eye conditions, we will review the major causes contributing to three bothersome eye concerns: dark circles, puffy eyes, and under eye wrinkles. Pinpointing the origin of these skin and contour issues guides us in selecting optimal treatment approaches.

Causes of Dark Circles

Dark circles can appear as a shadowy discoloration or dusky hue in the under eye region. Contributing factors include:

- Pigmentation - With aging, melanocyte cells may accumulate causing darker pigment to become visible through the thin undereye skin. Ethnicity, genetics, and sun exposure affect pigment production.

- Vascularization - Under eye veins and capillaries may become more visible as skin thins with age. Blood byproducts also accumulate causing darker discoloration.

- Shadow Effect - Descent or loosening of the tear trough ligament allows orbital fat pads to protrude forward, casting a shadow.

- Hollowness - Volume loss in the lower lid-cheek junction creates a sunken, darkened appearance.

- Lifestyle Factors - Lack of sleep, poor diet, dehydration, smoking, and alcohol use can exacerbate undereye darkening.

Clearly there are numerous intricately related factors driving the development of unappealing dark undereye circles. Targeted solutions will need to address pigmentation, vascularity, volume loss, and lifestyle habits for optimal rejuvenation.

Causes of Puffy Eyes

Puffiness around the eyes refers to swelling or protrusion causing visible fullness and bags under the eyes. Typical culprits behind puffy eyes include:

Fluid Retention - Allergies, genetics, sleep deprivation or fatigued eyes allow fluid accumulation around the periorbital area.

Structural Changes - Aging weakens connective tissue and muscles around the eyes allowing orbital fat pads to herniate forward.

Toxicity & Medications - Salt, alcohol, or medications lead to localized fluid retention and swelling under the eyes.

Medical Conditions - Diseases like thyroid dysfunction, kidney disease, or liver failure manifest in puffy eyes.

Increased Adiposity - Weight gain, water retention, and loose skin can cause puffy eyes and exacerbate other factors.

Clearly there is no single cause of bothersome under eye puffiness and bags. An intricate interplay of factors including inflammation, structural changes, toxins, disease and adiposity contribute in varying degrees. Customized treatment requires addressing the array of potential influences.

Causes of Under Eye Wrinkles

Wrinkles, fine lines, and crepey skin around the eyes develop gradually over time but have identifiable originating factors, including:

- Natural Aging - Skin loses elasticity, fat pads descend, bony prominence increases, and collagen/hyaluronic acid levels decline.

- Repetitive Expressions - Frequent animate facial expressions etch lines horizontally across the forehead and vertically between the brows. Squinting strains the outside corners.

13

- Sun Exposure - UV radiation generates free radicals, degrading supportive skin proteins like collagen and elastin. This accelerates aging.
- Genetics & Ethnicity - Some individuals have weaker undereye collagen and thinner skin prone to early wrinkling.
- Lifestyle Factors - Smoking, alcohol, poor sleep, dehydration, and high sugar intake degrade skin.

Clearly the development of eye wrinkles, much like circles and puffiness, is multifactorial. Customized solutions require addressing collagen support, skin protection, hydration, and lifestyle habits for smoother, firmer, more youthful eye contours.

Now that we recognize the major culprits behind circles, puffiness, and wrinkling we can thoughtfully develop treatment regimens targeting the various causal factors using principles of ocular health, structural enhancement, skin rejuvenation, and healthy lifestyle habits for dramatically improved eye aesthetics.

Eye Health and Aging

As we explore treatments to address concerns like dark circles, puffiness and wrinkles for more youthful-appearing eyes, we must consider normal age-related changes to eye health. Understanding the aging process allows us to differentiate normal vs. abnormal findings, set realistic expectations, and select proactive solutions for maintaining eye function.

External Eye Aging

External changes to the eyes and surrounding structures result from decades of repetitive animation, environmental exposure, decreased tissue elasticity, bone resorption, and fat pad descent. Key aging signs include:

- Wrinkles - Skin loses collagen support, elastin networks degrade, and cellular regeneration declines leading to wrinkles and crepey skin around the eyes.

- Volume Loss - Orbital fat pads sag, bony sockets expand, and cartilage shrinks. This structural descent creates hollowness and shadows.

- Dryness - Oil and tear production decreases while meibomian gland dysfunction increases, causing dry areas and irritation.

- Ectropion/Entropion - Horizontal lid laxity allows the eyelids to evert (ectropion) or invert (entropion) causing chronic irritation.

- Dermatochalasis - Excess, sagging eyelid skin develops, sometimes impairing peripheral vision.

Clearly time takes its toll on the integrity of structures supporting healthy eye function and youthful appearance. However, not all aging changes are unavoidable. Targeted solutions can proactively curb deterioration.

Internal Eye Aging

While external changes generally have more cosmetic impact, internal age-related changes can affect vision and ocular health. Common manifestations include:

- Presbyopia - The lenses lose elasticity and ability to accommodate focus on near objects due to lifelong protein crosslinking. Reading glasses become necessary.

- Cataracts - Denaturation, clumping and aggregation of lens proteins reduce transparency and obstruct light passage to the retina resulting in cloudy or blurry vision.

- Retinal Changes - The macula may accumulate waste pigment (drusen) leading to central visual deterioration or yellowed peripheral retina.

- Glaucoma - Age related narrowing and rigidity of aqueous outflow pathways causes increased intraocular pressure associated with gradual vision loss.
- Neurodegeneration - Retinal ganglion cell dysfunction and progressive loss of nerve connections impairs signaling to the brain leading to vision decline.

While surgery, glasses or medications can improve vision changes, prevention through nutrition and lifestyle optimization may curb degeneration and prolong healthy ocular function.

Maintaining Eye Health

Thankfully many age-related eye changes can be slowed through diligent self care:

- Consistent Eye Exams – Routine assessments by an eye doctor help detect subtle changes at early, more treatable stages.
- Nutrition - Antioxidants from fruits, vegetables and omega oils support cell health. Lutein, zeaxanthin and vitamins C and E protect the eyes.
- Hydration - Water intake preserves moisture in eye tissues and lubricating tear film.
- Sun Protection - Shielding eyes from UV exposure reduces free radical damage. Wide-brimmed hats add coverage.
- Targeted Eye Products - Using hydrating, replenishing eye creams, gels and serums preserves youthful appearance.
- Healthy Habits - Not smoking, maintaining ideal weight, regulating blood pressure and limiting alcohol intake help avoid ocular complications.

While intrinsic changes are inevitable, implementing proactive self-care from an early age can dramatically slow unsightly aging manifestations around the eyes for preserved function and aesthetics. Having covered anatomy, common issues, causation, and aging influences we now shift focus to solutions and treatments for rejuvenating the eye zone.

Assessing Your Eye Needs

Now that we have built a strong foundation exploring eye anatomy, common conditions, causes of specific concerns like circles and wrinkles, and influences of aging, we are ready to effectively evaluate our own eye health and aesthetic needs. Thorough self-assessment allows us to pinpoint priority areas and customize optimal treatment regimens.

Appearance Evaluation

First, analyze the appearance of your eye area checking for:

- Wrinkles & Fine Lines - Note wrinkle depth, length and location - crows feet, forehead lines, between brows. Are lines present even when face is relaxed?
- Crepiness & Skin Thinning - Inspect skin texture and translucency around eyes. Can underlying vessels be easily seen?
- Hyperpigmentation & Dark Circles - Check for brown patches or darkening. Does one side differ? Circle dark actual pigmented areas.
- Hollowness & Volume Loss - Assess fat pad protrusion and cheek-lid junction depth. Are skulls becoming more prominent under eyes?
- Puffiness, Bags & Undereye Circles - Outline the borders of any puffy, swollen areas using a colored pencil. Does puffiness fluctuate throughout day?

- Eyelid Changes - Inspect for skin excess, hooding, resting visibility of eyelid border or complete closure difficulties.
- Methodically evaluating appearance provides tangible visibility into which signs of aging are currently bothersome allowing us to pinpoint target areas for treatment.
- Symptom Analysis
- Beyond pure aesthetics, analyzing symptoms provides insight into functional issues affecting eye health:
- Dryness & Irritation - Note sensations of stinging, grittiness, pain indicating problems with lubrication.
- Vision Difficulties - Document issues with acuity fluctuations, glare, ghosting, double vision suggesting retinal issues.
- Eyestrain & Fatigue - Track headaches, soreness, intermittent blurriness that could stem from uncorrected refraction, improper ergonomics or screen overuse.
- Itching & Redness - Recurring irritation may indicate allergies or blepharitis.
- Excess Tearing - Watery eyes could signal infection, pore blockages or duct obstruction.

Monitoring symptoms provides vital clues on inflammatory conditions, surface problems, infections, or other processes requiring medical treatment before aesthetic concerns can be addressed.

Lifestyle Analysis

Certain lifestyle factors and daily habits greatly impact the health and aging of our eyes. Keep a journal tracking:

- Screen Use - Note total daily screen time for work and leisure across devices including phones, tablets, computers and TVs.

- Sleep Quantity & Quality - Document nightly sleep duration and sense of restedness upon waking. Lack of sleep is highly linked to eye puffiness and dark circles.

- Eye Strain Habits - Record ergonomics like screen height, distance, glare, font size, and work break frequency. Small adjustments can significantly improve strain.

- Contact Lens Wear - Track hours worn daily and meticulousness with case hygiene, lens replacement schedule and adherence to wearing restrictions.

- Sun Exposure - Detail hours spent outdoors without UV eye protection via hats, glasses or shields. Exposure greatly accelerates aging.

- Smoking & Alcohol Use - Quantify tobacco use and alcohol intake which degrade eye tissues.

Identifying lifestyle factors allows us to modify routines to support eye health and maximize outcomes from aesthetic eye rejuvenation treatments.

Consistently assessing our eye area appearance, symptoms, and habits provides tremendous insight into developing customized treatment regimens targeting current problem zones for significantly improved aesthetics and comfortable function.

Nutrition for Healthy Eyes

Proper nutrition plays a pivotal role in supporting eye health and function. Incorporating key antioxidants, vitamins, minerals, and healthy fats lays the foundation for clear vision, while simultaneously fighting factors that lead to circles, puffiness and wrinkles around the eyes. This section explores optimal dietary composition for reducing visible aging changes.

Antioxidants

Antioxidants counteract oxidative damage from free radicals that accumulate through sun exposure and metabolism. This prevents degradation of collagen and elastin proteins around the eyes. Beneficial antioxidant sources include:

- Vitamin C - Abundant in citrus fruits, berries, tomatoes, peppers and dark green vegetables. Boosts collagen synthesis.

- Vitamin E - Found in plant oils, nuts, seeds, whole grains, spinach and avocado. Protects cell membranes.

- Lutein & Zeaxanthin - Carotenoids concentrated in dark leafy greens like kale and spinach. Filter blue light and absorb UV rays in the eye.

- Beta-Carotene - Orange pigmented fruits and vegetables like carrots, pumpkin, sweet potato and squash. Maintains surface tissues.

- Bioflavonoids - Present in green tea, berries and citrus fruits. Prevent collagen breakdown and scavenge radicals.

Essential Vitamins

Certain vitamins play integral roles in eye cell metabolism and function:

Vitamin A - Supports corneal surface health and cell differentiation in the retina. Found in liver, fish oil, dairy products, and orange/green vegetables.

B Vitamins - Aid tissue repair and renewal. Sources include whole grains, meat, lentils, seeds and nuts.

Vitamin C - Promotes collagen structure stability defending against wrinkling and vasculature changes causing dark circles.

Vitamin D - Linked to reduced risk of macular degeneration and dry eyes. Synthesized from sunlight and found in fish oil, dairy and mushrooms.

Vitamin E - Protects delicate eye cell membranes from destruction by reactive oxygens species which drive aging changes.

Key Minerals & Electrolytes

Minerals serve as enzyme cofactors for critical chemical reactions in ocular tissues:

Zinc - Required for proper visual development and retinal function. Oysters and organ meats are rich sources.

Copper - Essential for crosslinking and stabilization of collagen networks supporting youthful skin structure. Found with zinc and iron foods.

Potassium - Vital for nerve signal transmission. Bananas, avocados, leafy greens and beans supply potassium.

Magnesium & Selenium - Aid glutathione production which is the eye's premier endogenous antioxidant, protecting delicate cells from damage leading to poor regulation of vascular changes around the eyes. High levels in spinach, nuts, legumes, and seafood.

Omega Fatty Acids - Support tear film lipid layer stability and guard against dryness. Best sourced from cold water fatty fish, flax and chia seeds.

Clearly nutritional composition has far reaching effects on the health, surface conditions, and visible aging changes around the vulnerable tissues surrounding our eyes. Conscientious dietary improvements initiate a cascade of beneficial cellular reactions that provide enhanced collagen support, free radical protection, hydration and microcirculation for dramatically improved aesthetic outcomes from topical eye treatments. Nutrition establishes a thriving internal ecosystem allowing rejuvenating products to optimize results.

Sleep and Eye Rejuvenation

Adequate sleep plays an integral role in eye health and rejuvenation. Sleep allows our body to repair tissues, remove waste byproducts, and restore energy levels. Limited sleep deprives eyes of this crucial biological recovery, accelerating visible aging changes like dark circles, undereye bags and wrinkles. Prioritizing healthy sleep hygiene lays the foundation for successfully treating eye area concerns.

Sleep Mechanisms

To understand the critical impacts of sleep deprivation, we must first understand intrinsic sleep processes. There are two primary phases:

Non-Rapid Eye Movement (NREM) - Consists of three progressive stages of light to deep sleep in which heart rate, respiration, and brain waves gradually decline.

Rapid Eye Movement (REM) - Characterized by darting eye movements behind closed lids, diminished muscle tone throughout the body, and activation of brain regions governing sight, movement, and dreams.

We cycle through NREM and REM phases multiple times during a typical night's sleep in order to recharge physical and cognitive functioning. Disrupting this cycling impedes restorative processes.

Impacts on Eyes

Missing sleep has pronounced effects on eye health and appearance manifesting as:

Bloodshot Eyes - Capillaries become dilated and inflamed from stress hormone and chemical increases during wakefulness deprivation. This gives the whites of eyes a diffusely red, irritated look.

Puffy Eyes & Bags - Fluid accumulation results from compromised lymphatic drainage pathways which normally filter extracellular fluid during sleep cycles. Excess fluid pools around eyes.

Dark Circles - Continued metabolism without cell renewal causes waste pigment byproducts like bilirubin to accumulate under eyes giving a darker, shadowed look.

Dry Eyes - Critical tear production and turnover rebalances during REM cycles. Short changing sleep causes imbalance in tear volume and chemical composition leading to irritation.

Wrinkles - Collagen production peaks during late NREM sleep when cell division and repair occurs. Inadequate sleep hampers collagen development, accelerating aging.

Clearly dark circles, puffiness, dryness and wrinkles can signal suboptimal sleep quantity or efficiency. Making sleep a priority is essential for eye revitalization.

Optimizing Sleep Habits

Implementing healthy sleep hygiene rituals bolsters rejuvenating REM and NREM cycling leading to improved undereye appearance and ocular function:

Consistency - Maintain fixed bed and wake times including weekends to properly calibrate circadian cycles and cue tiredness.

Wind Down Ritual - Spend 30 minutes screening down lights, devices, mental activities. Take a bath, sip herbal tea, stretch gently.

Comfort - Invest in supportive pillows and mattresses. Keep bedroom cool, clean and quiet to limit disturbance. Consider blackout curtains.

Supplementation - Discuss melatonin, magnesium or antihistamine use short term if having difficulty relaxing into sleep.

Stimulant Curtailment - Avoid caffeine, large meals, alcohol or vigorous evening exercise disrupting sleep cycles.

Healthy sleep empowers vigorous eye rejuvenation capabilities through enhanced collagen development, waste clearance, fluid regulation, and tear production. Prioritize nightly sleep consistency as the cornerstone for combating puffy tired looking eyes.

Managing Stress and Fatigue

Our modern, connected lives subject eyes to near constant stimulation and demands for attention. Chronic stress and visual overload tires the eyes, manifesting in aesthetic concerns like dark undereye circles, bags, and wrinkles. Effectively managing fatigue and stress is essential for revitalized eyes.

Ocular Impacts

Eye strain and fatigue have pronounced impacts on appearance and comfort including:

- Muscle Strain - Persistent squinting and repetitive animation etch lines at the outside eye corners and between brows leading to a worried, weary look.

- Vascular Congestion - Stress triggers release of hormones like cortisol and epinephrine which increase blood pressure. This causes blood vessels around eyes to swell and darken.

- Inflammation - Tired eyes release inflammatory cytokines generating puffiness and bags under eyes along with redness.

- Dryness - Intense visual effort reduces blinking leading to tear film instability, irritation, and compensatory watering.

- Wrinkling - Frequent muscle contractions degrade supporting collagen while eyestrain flattens protective orbital fat pads causing crepey wrinkled skin.

Clearly the visible tolls of eye exhaustion are extensive but strategic management to reduce fatigue and tension can reclaim a more vibrant wide-eyed appearance.

Assessing Eye Strain

Recognizing personal symptoms of eye strain empowers us to modify aggravating habits and environments. Track intensity of:

Headaches - Temple tension, sinus pressure behind eyes signal eyestrain.

Blurry Vision - Difficulty shifting or maintaining clear near focus hints overworked eye muscles.

Eye Discomfort - Sensations of stinging, burning or grit in eyes indicate irritation, inflammation and dryness.

Light Sensitivity - Glare, halos and difficulties with night vision stem from photoreceptor exhaustion.

Double Vision - Misaligned images point to extraocular muscle imbalance from near work repetition.

Reducing Fatigue Triggers

Customizing changes based on our strain profile can dramatically improve eye vigor, comfort and aesthetics:

20-20-20 Rule - Every 20 minutes during screen tasks look up 20 feet away for 20 seconds to rest eyes.

Proper Posture - Position screens at level eye height and 18-30 inches away to minimize squinting and effort.

Lighting - Reduce overhead glare with diffused lighting. Avoid working in dim environments prompting eyes to overwork.

Computer Specs - Increase display resolution, adjust font sizes for easier reading without continual focusing adaptation. Blue light filtering lenses help ease adaptation between tasks.

Lubricating Eye Drops - Rehydrating irritated eyes improves stamina and reduces inflammatory damage leading to aesthetic issues over time.

With some adjustments to minimize sources of eye exhaustion, we can protect delicate tissues from wear and tear which drive visible aging changes around the eyes. Supportive environment and habits reduce demands on extraocular muscles and dryness prompting improved lubrication, circulation and collagen support for restored vibrancy.

Exercises for Tired Eyes

Targeted eye exercises and facial massage techniques can dramatically relieve eye strain when incorporated regularly into our routines. By gently working the ocular muscles and stimulating circulation, exercises boost oxygenation removing inflammatory waste byproducts that induce fatigue puffiness and darkening. Here we explore easy, effective exercises to revitalize eyes.

Rotations

Simple eye rotations effectively stretch extraocular muscles stressed from repetitive near focus. rotation exercises include:

Palming - Rub hands vigorously together to stimulate warmth and circulation. Cup palms gently over closed eyes without applying pressure. Allow eyes to relax while sensing palms. Palming provides soothing darkness reducing strain.

Horizontal Rotations - Sit comfortably looking straight ahead. Rotate eyes smoothly side to side focusing on finger movement at maximum left and right eccentricities. Repeat 10 times.

Vertical Rotations - Perform up and down rotations following fingertip movement highest and lowest with eyes while keeping head still. Complete 10 repetitions.

Diagonal Rotations - Trace fingertip diagonally down-right, then up-left such that eyes follow in opposite direction concentrating on full range diagonal motion. Repeat 5 times per diagonal.

Rotations realign muscle balance, stimulate fluid drainage from circulating lymphatics, and instill awareness of tension buildup so we can consciously release eye strain throughout the day.

Press Compressions

Applying mild digital pressure around the eyes helps pump excess fluids trapped in surrounding loose tissues to improve fatigue puffiness, bags and dark circles:

Orbital Massage - With relaxed fingertips gently massage the complete bone orbit of each eye pressing inward and outward 10 times. Avoid directly touching the globes themselves.

Lower Lid Compression - Lightly grip the skin just below lower lashes between index fingers and thumbs. Pull down gently before sliding fingers out toward ears 10 times per side to release fluid buildup.

Upper Lid Compression - Similarly grasp each upper lid at the lash line gently pinching and sliding outwardly above the brows 10 times to stimulate drainage.

Bridge Compression - Use knuckles to apply gentle inward pressure at the inner corners nearest bridge of nose and slide knuckles outward along brows to temples 10 times.

Compressive manual techniques improve circulatory and lymphatic clearing of inflammatory waste byproducts that create the look of chronically fatigued eyes.

Stress Relief

Since mental strain and worry translates into physical eye tension, relaxing through mindfulness breaks prevents chronic squinting, scowling and furrowing which etch lines over years:

Breath Focusing - Close eyes. Inhale slowly visualizing breathing in calmness. Exhale purposefully expelling stress. Repeat five breath cycles allowing shoulders to sink down.

Guided Imagery - Visualize a serene comforting place like lying lakeside or wandering through a spring meadow. Engage senses enjoying flowers, gentle noises, cool breezes. Allow worries to float away.

Daily eye self-massage and stress relief through purposeful relaxation provides the overworked windows to our world a much needed break from continual bombardment. Just five minutes twice daily over weeks and months promotes revitalization helping turn back the clock on puffiness, wrinkling and shadows.

Screen Time and Your Eyes

In our modern world, screens in the form of phones, tablets, computers and televisions pervade nearly every moment of our waking lives. While these devices improve connectivity, entertainment and efficiency, chronic gazing at artificially lit displays fatigues our eyes accelerating visible aging changes like dark circles, under eye bags and wrinkling over years. Optimizing device use preserves our peepers.

Digital Eye Strain

Prolonged staring at bright, pixelated screens strains the eyes in various ways leading to irritation, inflammation and tissue damage:

Focus Fatigue - Screens lie at fixed close focal points requiring sustained accommodation and convergence instead of regular distance refocusing which is more natural. Ciliary muscles tire.

Reduced Blinking - Engrossed digital viewers blink far less frequently allowing tear film to evaporate and eyes to dry out, especially with exposure to unblinking blue light emitting devices.

Disruption of Circadian Rhythm - Light emitted suppresses natural melatonin release and disrupts sleep cycles impeding essential biological repair.

Oxidative Stress - High energy visual light rays generate free radicals bombarding delicate eye cell structures gradually degrading collagen integrity supporting youthful plump form. Chronic digital eye strain stresses structures and impedes restorative downtime for fluid regulation and tissue rebuilding - changes become etched in fine lines, dark shadows and chronic redness over time.

Optimizing Screen Use

Thankfully minor adjustments in our screen habits can dramatically alleviate eye strain and visible damage:

20-20-20 Rule - Every 20 minutes using screens look up 20 feet away for 20 seconds which relieves focusing muscles.

Proper Positioning - Position screens 18-28 inches directly facing eyes with top just below eye level to minimize exposure and accommodation demands.

Ambient Lighting - Keep room lighting brighter than screens to reduce pupil dilation and effort. Use bias lighting behind screens.

Increase Text Size - Enlarge fonts and interfaces on devices to make content more visible and readable without squinting strain.

Blue Light Filtering - Enable nightshift device settings or wear tinted computer glasses to block highest energy blue emissions for improved sleep.

Small adjustments to our digital habits improve eye ergonomics, visual efficiency and downstream health. Preserving eyes against tech fatigue improves visibility of screens themselves while maintaining that bright, wide-eyed glow signifying youthfulness and vitality over our lifespan.

Eye Creams and Serums

Specialized eye creams and serums deliver targeted ingredients to the delicate skin surrounding our eyes to hydrate, nourish and rejuvenate this thinnest skin of the body, combating fine lines, wrinkles, dark circles and puffiness. Applying formulations designed specifically for the eye region optimizes absorption and effectiveness for dramatically improved appearance.

Benefits

The thinner dermal layer around our eyes lacks sebaceous oil glands and has less subcutaneous fat cushioning so the area requires specialized care. Using dedicated creams and serums provides:

Hydration - Rich moisturizing ingredients in eye formulations hydrate surface skin cells and support deeper structures to plump, providing a more youthful cushion.

Peptides & Growth Factors - These stimulate collagen and elastin production in the delicate eye area targeting fine lines and crepiness.

Lightening Ingredients - Compounds like vitamin C, kojic acid, and liquorice root extract address pigmentation changes contributing to dark undereye shadows and spotting.

Anti-Inflammatories - Calming botanical extracts, vitamins, and oils soothe irritated puffy eyes exacerbated by allergies, sleeplessness, and strain.

Caffeine Constriction - Applied to fat cells, caffeine in products stimulates drainage pathways decreasing fluid accumulation leading to puffy eyes and undereye bags.

Formula Selection

With countless eye creams cluttering the marketplace making selection overwhelming, focus needs on finding products matching individual eyes' needs and concerns like:

Dryness Relief - Seek thick moisturizing balms containing hydrating ceramides, plant oils and shea butter. Layer a serum underneath.

Puffiness & Bags - Caffeine-based gels with gentle diuretic extracts like green tea help relieve excess fluid accumulation and fat protrusion. Use gentle tapping application motions.

Dark Circles & Shadows - Brightening formulations feature vitamin C, kojic acid, retinol, niacinamide and peptides to improve pigmentation and strengthen thin skin.

Wrinkles & Fine Lines- Collagen-stimulating products with hyaluronic acid, amino peptide complexes, antioxidants and ceramides refortify suppleness and smoothness.

With routine daily use, dedicated eye potions provide transformative improvements in fighting fine lines for wide-awake, vibrant aesthetic outcome.

Application Tips

Proper application maximizes eye cream absorption and effectiveness:

Light Massage - Use delicate ring fingertips to gently tap and press products around the orbital bone working from inner corners along lashlines outward to temples.

Hydrate Lower Lids - Ensure creams contact delicate lower lid skin and the often neglected lateral hollows adjacent the nose where deepening tear troughs lead to darkened shadows.

Serum Layering - Apply watery serums with potent actives before heavier moisturizing creams for enhanced penetration. The thinner serum hydrates allowing better cream absorption.

Set with Powder - After allowing creams to absorb fully, set lids with a mineral powder to limit product creeping into eyes throughout the day.

Using professional quality eye serums and creams specifically developed for the delicate eyes and lids goes a tremendous way to reversing environmental aging damage over years for restored radiance. With some guidance on optimal ingredient selection and application technique, results can prove dramatic.

Botanical Treatments

Botanical extracts derived from herbs, roots, flowers and nutrients rich plants provide a powerful way to nourish delicate tissues around eyes plagued with fine lines, dark circles and bagginess without harsh chemicals. Botanicals' bioactive phytonutrients strengthen skin resilience while eliminating inflammation and pigmentation. This section highlights optimal botanicals.

Soothing Botanicals

Botanicals like chamomile, cucumber, aloe vera and green tea deliver calming, hydrating antioxidants to appease irritated under eyes:

Chamomile - Contains matricaria phytochemicals like chamazulene having anti-inflammatory, antibacterial and skin healing benefits to reverse puffiness and redness.

Cucumber - Cucumis sativus fruit extract, vitamins and minerals cool inflammation, stimulate collagen and serves as an anti-wrinkle antioxidant fighting free radicals from UV exposure and sleep deprivation byproducts which accumulate in tissues.

Aloe Vera - glycoproteins and polysaccharides in aloe boost hyaluronic acid improving skin moisture retention and suppleness while other compounds reduce tyrosinase enzyme activity correcting pigmentation.

Green Tea - Polyphenolic compounds called catechins stimulate blood flow to clear toxic inflammatory mediators through the thin eye skin revealing brighter skin and eyes. EGCG fights collagen breakdown.

These ancient botanicals offer wellspring of reparative and protective nutrients helping optimize the eye environ.

Stimulatory Botanicals

Beyond anti-inflammatory calmatives, some botanicals provide stimulation to increase collagen development essential for combating crepey wrinkles:

Ginseng - Ginsenosides in Korean red ginseng energize dermal fibroblasts to synthesize more supportive collagen fibers while improving microcirculation. This builds firmness defending against wrinkling.

Ginkgo Biloba - Ginkgo flavonoids protect blood vessels supporting microcapillaries around the eyes to reduce leakage contributing to shadows and darkness while the terpenoids enhance tone.

Horse Chestnut - Aescin compounds strengthen venous walls while decreasing capillary permeability preventing blood byproducts from accumulating under eyes. This reduces dark hues.

Butcher's Broom - Ruscogenin stimulates veins assisting drainage to reduce localized blood pooling while anti-elastases preserve supportive proteins keeping lids and surrounding skin firm.

Botanicals' breadth of benefits for eye aesthetics through anti-inflammatory relief complemented by collagen boosting for fortified smoothness makes them core additions to topical rejuvenation regimens.

Botanical extracts are sensitizing alone so combine into gel or lotions. Standard application guidelines apply:

Perform Patch Test - Dab small amount on inner forearm watching for redness or itching which indicate potential sensitivity.

Use Gentle Motions - Lightly pat serums or creams containing botanicals around the delicate eye zone using ring fingers for thin skin protection.

Appropriate Frequency - Begin applying botanical eye formulations just once every few days then gradually build tolerance to daily use for optimal reparative results over weeks and months.

Thoughtfully formulated botanicals promote eye revitalization from the inside out by optimizing the local environment, fuelling essential structures, and protecting against further insult. Notice the difference botanicals make in combating fine lines, puffiness and dark shadows.

Vitamins and Minerals

Vitamins and minerals serve as vital cofactors and enzyme components supporting essential biological processes in ocular tissues that preserve youthful eye aesthetics over years. Deficiencies manifest in accelerated aging changes. Optimizing intake through nutrition and supplementation lays firm foundation.

Key Vitamins

Certain vitamins have pronounced impacts on visible eye revitalization:

Vitamin A - Protects delicate mucous membranes around eyes while promoting cell growth needed for continual skin renewal keeping lids looking fresh instead of weathered.

Vitamin C - Critical for collagen production providing firmness and smoothness. Antioxidant properties defend connective tissue proteins around eyes against UV degradation to maintain vibrant appearance over decades.

Vitamin E - Prevents cell membrane damage induced by stress oxidative species from eyestrain and environmental exposure which eat away at collagen integrity leading to wrinkling and laxity. Potent antioxidant protects youthful land delicate eye structures.

Vitamin K - Reduces vascular fragility and leakage preventing blood byproducts from accumulating in thin orbital undereye skin hiding veins causing darkening and shadows characteristic of vitamin deficiency.

Regular intake through food sources combines with selective topical application via serums to optimize eye zone revitalization capabilities.

Key Minerals

Minerals like copper and zinc enable hundreds of enzymes driving essential reactions:

Zinc - Structural component for enzymes regulating cell division supporting continual renewal of delicate eyelid tissues. Deficiency causes visible skin atrophy. Protects fats cushioning eyes from free radical damage which ages.

Copper - Required for crosslinking of fibrous collagen and elastin networks providing firm tensile support woven throughout eye muscles and surrounding skin. Critical mineral keeps eyes lifted.

Selenium - Component of glutathione peroxidase enzymes neutralizing free radicals stemming from eyestrain and sun exposure which degrade collagen plumpness leading to wrinkling. Boosts tissue recovery.

Magnesium - Calms nervous activity to relax near constant muscle tension from squinting and worry which etches fine lines around eyes. Relaxation supports youthful rested appearance.

Adequate mineral presence enables proper enzymatic function protecting delicate eye region from processes driving aging changes like wrinkling, dark circles, and irritation.

Thoughtful supplementation alongside food sources insures we get enough of these critical micronutrients given essential roles in defending eye integrity and aesthetics despite frequent depletion from stressors of modern living. Supporting healthy eyes happens from the inside out!

Anti-inflammatory Ingredients

Inflammation underlies many aesthetic eye concerns like puffiness, bags, dark circles, and redness. Allergic reactions, sleep deprivation, eye strain, and repetitive muscle movements trigger inflammatory cascades around the eyes. Applying targeted ingredients with anti-inflammatory effects can dramatically calm irritation to improve appearance.

Key Ingredients

Many cosmeceutical ingredients like botanical oils and antioxidants have soothing, anti-inflammatory properties:

Arnica - Arnica Montana flower extract includes inflammatory-blocking sesquiterpene lactones that reduce edema, bruising, and allergic reactions leading to puffy eyes and redness. Improves circulation.

Jojoba Oil - Mimics skin's sebum to reinforce skin barrier function protecting against irritant penetration leading to inflammatory water retention and puffiness. Contains anti-inflammatory tocopherols.

Aloe Vera - Mucilaginous polysaccharides coat and protect while amino acids soothe irritated eye area tissue caused by environmental insults. Reduces cytokine release.

Green Tea Extract-Polyphenolic catechins like epigallocatechin gallate (EGCG) inhibit release inflammation-driving enzymes like collagen-destroying matrix metalloproteinases minimizing fine lines and oxidative damage from UV light exposure and blue light overuse.

Caffeine - Constricts blood vessels to decrease fluid accumulation while suppressing prostaglandins and interleukins normally released during the inflammatory response to allergens or eyestrain.

Thoughtfully formulated anti-inflammatory eye creams can make a significant difference reducing visible redness, puffiness, and irritation over time through daily application.

Mechanisms of Action

These beneficial ingredients influence multiple levels of the inflammatory cascade:

Cooling Vasoconstriction - Caffeine and plant extracts like horse chestnut, butcher's broom and ginkgo biloba narrow blood vessels to decrease leakage of fluid and inflammatory mediators. This reduces edema and puffiness.

Blocking Histamine - Allergic reactions release histamine triggering vasodilation, itching and increased vascular permeability resulting swelling. Arnica, aloe and green tea bioactives prevent histamine binding reducing allergy symptoms.

Hindering Prostaglandins - Jojoba oil, chamomile and caffeine slow production of pain and inflammation propagating prostaglandins that increase cytokine production which chews away at structural collagen integrity.

Preventing Transudation - Fortifying veins and lymphatics with botanical extracts like gotu kola prevents leakage of fluid, proteins and cells into surrounding tissues preventing bags and puffiness characteristic of irritation.

Using eye care products with these natural anti-inflammatory helpers promotes eyes which look and feel less irritated, overtired and shadowed from perpetual assault by environmental and digital threats seeking to degrade delicate eye tissues.

Considerations

When applying anti-inflammatory eye ingredients take precautions:

Conduct Patch Test - Dab ingredients on skin assessing for redness or itching indicating potential sensitivity before applying near eyes.

Use Appropriate Frequency - Start applying anti-inflammatory eye products once every few days then gradually increase to daily for optimal effects once sensitivity is ruled out.

Pair Oral Antihistamines - Supplementing topicals with temporary oral antihistamines offsets allergy driven inflammation during high pollen seasons.

Controlling eye inflammation protects delicate collagen networks and microvasculature nourishing eyes to retain that vibrant, rested glow associated with youth. Make anti-inflammatory ingredients core component of eye care routines.

Retinoids and Retinol

Among the most researched skincare ingredients proven to stimulate collagen production, retinoids - like over-the-counter retinol and prescription strength retinoic acid - rank among the most efficacious anti-aging compounds. Retinoids renew skin by boosting cell turnover revealing fresher layers. Harnessing their power rejuvenates eye aesthetics.

Mechanisms

The vitamin A derivative retinoic acid binds specialized receptors called RARs and RXRs on the DNA within skin cells to boost gene transcription and modulation of processes like:

Collagen Synthesis - Activation of messenger proteins increases output from fibroblast cells that produce supporting collagen proteins maintaining firm flexible skin resistant to wrinkling and crepiness.

Cell Turnover - Accelerating conversion of old damaged surface skin cells into younger viable layers gives improved tone and coloration. Evens irregular pigmentation deposited in tired looking under eye hollows.

Skin Thickness - Direct stimulation of elastin and glycosaminoglycans production plumps dermal layers protecting eyes from crinkling while improving barrier functionality.

In essence, retinoids turn back the clock on visible aging changes to eye area skin revealing refreshed, youthful aesthetics.

Forms

Retinoids exist in various strength formulations based on conversion requirements:

Retinoic Acid - The directly usable retinoid form binds cellular receptors without conversion Required for prescription strengths. Brand names include Retin-A, Renova, Tazorac.

Retinaldehyde - This aldehyde form undergoes one conversion step to transform into retinoic acid. Found in some over the counter night creams.

Retinol - The alcohol requires enzymatic conversion to retinaldehyde then retinoic acid for activity. Available in many OTC serums, gels and eye products at concentrations up to 2%.

Using appropriately formulated retinoid eye products targets improved collagen density, elasticity, even tone and smoothed texture for restored youthfulness.

Best Practices

Responsibly incorporating these powerful victors harnesses benefits while avoiding irritation and redness:

Start Low Strength - Begin with 0.25% - 0.5% OTC retinol checking sensitivity before gradually working percentage upwards week-by-week to improve tolerance allowing fuller reparative effects.

Buffer if Sensitive - Mix pea sized amount with gentle moisturizer when applying to sensitive areas like eye zone as buffer until skin adjusts. Reduces dryness and flaking.

Alternate Nights Initially - Apply retinoid eye product every second or third evening as skin builds resilience. Allows recovery preventing redness.

Supportive Regimen - Pair with antioxidant serums to reduce any photosensitivity. Always apply SPF 30+ sunscreen during day.

Leveraging anti-aging might of retinoids with responsible application optimizes improvements to eye wrinkling, pigmentation and dullness issues stemming from intrinsic skin changes over decades. Proven weapon against chronic challenges of time and environment. Handle with care!

Chapter Four

Spa-Like Treatments

Applying cold compresses, cool gel packs, chilled eye masks and even cucumber slices cools inflammation to relieve puffy eyes, dark circles and bags. The vasoconstrictive effects of cold therapy constrict blood vessels, improve drainage and reduce swelling. Consistent cold treatment eases multiple factors causing tired eyes.

Reducing Puffiness

The anti-inflammatory and vasoconstrictive properties of cold application targets puffiness in various ways:

Narrows Blood Vessels - The drop in temperature causes vessels to temporarily constrict allowing less fluid and blood to leak into surrounding tissues. This deflates puffiness and plumps hollow tear troughs.

Slows Cellular Metabolism - Chilling skin tissues decreases activity levels and metabolic demands. Cells produce fewer waste inflammatory metabolites that manifest as swelling and circles.

Stimulates Lymphatic Drainage - Cold causes lymphatic vessels to contract more forcefully pumping excess proteins and fluids pooled around eyes through filtration nodes. This evacuates bags.

Prevents Histamine Release - Stabilizing mast cells with cold prevents inflammatory immune cells from releasing histamine and cytokines prompting swelling cascade seen with allergies and sleeplessness.

Routine cold therapy trains blood vessels and lymphatics improving tone and drainage competency to reverse puffy eyes.

Optimizing Cold Treatment

Certain methods and durations provide optimal rejuvenating effects:

Cucumber Slices - Chilled cucumber applied directly beneath eyes not only cools but delivers astringent cucurbitacins and antioxidants to treat irritation. Slice fresh cucumbers storing in fridge for quick use.

Cool Compresses - Soak clean soft washcloth in ice water, wring out then apply gently over closed eyes for 5-10 minutes allowing cooling sensation to penetrate tissue. Re-chill cloth as needed.

Gel Bead Masks - Specialized eye masks with built-in gel beads maintain consistent cooling for 10-15 minutes without dripping. This hands free option conforms around eye contours for concentrated effects.

Posture - Lean back while applying cold therapy allowing gravity to assist drainage. Gently massaging tissue from inner to outer corners further enhances fluid evacuation.

Consistent cold treatment trains tissues improving tone and drainage while thwarting inflammation development responsible for bags and puffiness leaving eyes looking refreshed and wide awake.

Precautions

Take care when applying any temperature extreme near vision organs:

Avoid Direct Contact - Don't allow chilled implements to directly contact eye surface as extreme temperature shifts stress delicate corneas risking damage. Keep compresses just adjacent lids.

Limit Treatment Times - Start with brief 5 minutes building to not over 15 consecutive minutes to prevent rebound vasodilation response once cold is removed bringing fluids and blood rushing back.

Discontinue if Uncomfortable - Any sharp pain indicates ice burn potential. Numbness feeling is normal but intense stinging suggests withdrawal to prevent frostbite.

Listen to skin's cues and avoid direct globe contact when leveraging power of cold therapy for combating chronic puffiness or circles marring bright, vibrant eye aesthetics. Discover this soothing, refreshing remedy.

Hot and Warm Compresses

Heat application helps revitalize fatigued eyes plagued with puffiness and dark circles by boosting circulation, stimulating collagen renewal, easing muscle tension and promoting drainage. Alternating warm and cool therapy leverages benefits of temperature extremes for eye rejuvenation.

Improving Blood Flow

Applying heat expands blood vessels increasing local circulation while extravascular compression forces stagnant blood back into motion:

Vasodilation - Heat sensitive TRPV channels open prompting nitric oxide release which relaxes vessel walls. This brings fresh oxygenated blood to eye tissues and carries away waste. Improved perfusion reduces shadows.

Extravascular Compression - Heat swells extracellular matrix compressing vessels. Pressure gradient propels deoxygenated blood forward combating stasis which accumulates byproducts contributing to dark tinge in under eye hollows and along lash lines.

Lymph Flow - Expanding vessels creates bidirectional pull stimulating contracting lymph vessels to drain excess proteins and fluids held in tissues causing puffiness and bags. Warmth flowing into lymphatics prevents backflow.

Increasing blood and lymph circulation reverses appearing signs of fatigue caused by waste buildup and stagnation while delivering nutrients needed for tissue repair and collagen rebuilding critical to maintaining supple form.

Heat Effects

Beyond circulation enhancement, applied warmth exerts additional restorative effects:

Supports Immune Cells - Warming eye tissues spikes activity of macrophages, neutrophils and lymphocytes responsible for removing damaged cells and fighting infection protecting delicate mucosa from insult which degrades plumpness.

Boosts Cell Metabolism - Heat accelerates enzymatic reactions powering critical tissue repair pathways involving protein synthesis and waste product removal rejuvenating tired eyes from the inside out.

Stimulates Collagen Production - Warmth activates heat shock proteins which signal fibroblasts to increase output of supportive collagen fibers maintaining structure compromised by repeated animation strain etched in fine lines with age.

Relaxes Muscles - Soothing ocular muscles chronically contracted to focus near work or squint in glare relieves tension built up over years that allows rested eyes to open wider appearing more vibrant.

Methodology

Various modalities leverage warming benefits:

Warm Washcloth - Soak clean soft cotton towel in hot water, wring thoroughly then apply over closed lids for 5 minutes allowing conductive heat to penetrate and stimulate tissues. Reheat as needed.

Hydrogel Bead Mask - Specialized eye masks with builtin hydrogel beads release soothing warmth. Conforms to lids and sockets for handsfree directed treatment to melt away puffiness.

Dry Heat - Microwavable fabric packs, rice socks and buckwheat hull eye pillows emit gentle radiative dry heat. Unique alternative option avoiding moisture.

Combined Therapy - Alternate 5 minutes warm compresses followed by 5 minutes cool cloths to maximize vaso-pumping effects which push fluid buildup out of orbital tissues reversing bags and swelling.

Restorative warmth supports proper circulation and drainage essential to well-rested eyes. The radiant results speak for themselves. Rediscover this soothing, effective treatment.

Lymphatic Drainage Massages

The lymphatic system serves as the body's drainage network filtering excess proteins, waste products and fluids that accumulate in the spaces between cells and tissues. Stagnation of lymphatic drainage around the eyes manifests as unsightly puffiness, dark circles and bags. Gentle lymphatic massage techniques assist flow.

Lymphatic Basics

Unlike the circulatory system with an active pumping heart, the lymphatic system relies on intrinsic contractions of lymph vessels along with adjacent skeletal muscle movements and pressure gradients to propel lymph fluid through nodes before emptying into veins.

Around the eyes, multiple lymph nodes cluster near ear canal openings, along the neck and chest. Delicate vessels gather fluids and proteins leaked from fragile orbital capillaries pooling blood in loose undereye tissues. Restoring normal flow reduces localized edema.

Massage Benefits

Manual lymphatic drainage massage around the eyes helps:

Open Primary Vessels - Using light skin stretching strokes opens initial lymphatic capillaries allowing fluid entry so stagnant proteins can transport through collector vessels. These feed nodes.

Stimulate Contraction - Gentle pumping pressure followed by release mimics the contract-relax cycle experienced during muscle movements or breathing which naturally pumps lymph along filling channels.

Enhance Drainage - Tracing drainage paths with fingertips guides excess fluids trapped in head tissues down through nodes near collar bones toward venous return points improving apparent puffiness.

Reduce Congestion - Dispersing localized fluid pockets and thickened proteins concentrated around eyes decreases tissue density allowing improved perfusion of arteries and veins to nourish cells with oxygen.

Manual techniques reinforce intrinsic lymphatic flow disrupted through modern sedentary lifestyles. Restoration of eye lymphatic drainage reveals refreshed aesthetics.

Massage Techniques

Specialized movements target eye puffiness and dark circles:

Orbital Bone massage - Use fingertips to trace orbital bones above and below eyes gently pressing along borders to stimulate fluid movement from congested lacrimal glands outward through vessels circling the orbits.

Compression Pump - Place index and middle fingers directly under eyes sideways. Gently pinch skin outward toward ears then release. Repeat pinching motion 10 times using very light pressure to pump fluids through collectors.

Lymphatic Path Tracing - Lightly trace skin centripetally from outer upper cheekbones inward toward nose, under eyes and down sides of neck to coax stuck proteins and liquid down normal drainage paths.

Forehead Clear - Use palm to gently stretch forehead skin up then make small circular movements across entire forehead to disperse fluid before sweeping down temple and sides of nose clearing egressed proteins.

Be patient and consistent using a light touch. Daily eye lymphatic drainage regimens reshape dermal contours revealing bright wide awake eyes full of youth.

Botanical Eye Masks

Applying masks with potent plant-derived bioactive ingredients provides targeted delivery of vitamins, minerals, peptides and phytonutrients directly to the thin undereye skin to correct discoloration, puffiness and early wrinkling. Custom homemade blends and commercial formulations harness botanicals.

Primary Botanicals

Eye-rejuvenating masks show efficacy using the following thoughtfully combined dried herbs, powders and extracts:

Green Tea - Powerful antioxidants called catechins stimulate circulation, constrict blood vessels and rejuvenate skin cells reversing signs of aging like wrinkles, dull tone and sagging lids. Provides anti-inflammatory, antimicrobial support while improving texture.

Ginkgo Biloba - Ginkgo contains antioxidant compounds called flavonoids which strengthen capillaries around the eyes to prevent leakage and accumulation of byproducts which cause darkness. Terpenoids improve microcirculation revealing brighter eyes.

Chamomile - Calming vitamins and volatile oils from chamomile flowers relieve irritation and puffiness caused by environmental allergens or lack of sleep. Lightens skin.

Cucumber - Vitamins, minerals and astringent cucurbitacin glycosides in cucumber soothe, cool, and constrict blood vessels around eyes diminishing puffiness and shadows characteristic of poor drainage. Antioxidants prevent future damage.

Aloe Vera - Mucilaginous gel from aloe vera leaves coats, hydrates and protects thin under eye skin. Contains polysaccharides and hormones stimulating collagen fibers reducing fine lines with direct contact.

These safe, botanically-derived aids provide symptomatic relief reversing visible aging around the delicate eye contour when concentrated into masks.

Benefits

Routine application from homemade or retail botanical eye masks supply:

Targeted Delivery - Direct topical application maximizes absorption of beneficial vitamins and phytonutrients deeper into thin orbital tissues unlike passive creams. Concentrated actives tackle root aging causes.

Collagen Stimulation - Vitamin C, flavonoids, polysaccharides and plant hormones in ingredients prompt fibroblast cells to produce more collagen improving crepey skins.

Improved Vascular & Lymph Flow - Natural plant chemicals prompt mild vasoconstriction around eyes improving venous and lymphatic drainage reversing dark circles and bags.

Under Eye Brightening - Anti-inflammatory chamomile, antioxidant catechins and gingko clear stagnation to nourish and renew eye area cells reversing dullness. Lightens shadows.

Administration Tips

To optimize botanical masks:

Use Proper Mixing Ratios - Limit masks to 20% or less dried herb weight into paste or gel avoiding irritation. Start with 10% mixes then gradually increase concentration with repeated use for desired benefit intensity.

Chill Before Application - Cooling masks before applying boosts vasoconstriction. Place coats or sheet masks with botanical serum into fridge for 30+ minutes then relax applying over closed eyes for full 15-20 minutes. The cold and botanical combo provides eye rejuvenation.

Rinse Afterwards - Gently cleanse off botanical mask remnants after recommended time avoiding residue contact with cornea if any seeps upwards interfering with vision or ocular health.

Custom botanical formulas bring spa effectiveness home. Discover how these ancient plants support total eye revitalization revealing your eyes magnificent beauty.

Soothing Eye Patches

Specialized skin-toning eye gels and collagen masks provide a barrier supporting absorption of concentrated skin-restoring ingredients. Nutrient-rich patches combat fine lines, swelling, creping and discoloration. Consistent multi-modal patch formulas transform eye aesthetics.

Types of Eye Patches

A variety of time-release transdermal under eye patches target specific needs:

Soothing Skin Protectants - Gel or fabric patches containing calming botanicals like aloe vera, chamomile and cucumber relieve irritation to accelerate healing after cosmetic procedures while protecting thin skin against friction.

Eye Lift - Elastin and collagen-based biocellulose stickers cling tightly to cultivate mild compression smoothing creases while adhesive pull lifts drooping lids providing temporary rejuvenative effects until muscles relax post-removal.

Puffy Eye Reducers - Depuffing patches infuse skin with caffeine, ginger root, arnica and cold therapy beads to restrict dilated vessels, move lymphatic buildup and facilitate drainage reducing bags.

Dark Circle Faders - Brightening vitamin C, licorice root and kojic or hyaluronic acid ampoules reduce pigmentation and hollowness for gradual, cumulative lightening of dark under eye circles with routine use.

Specialized patches provide immediate cosmetic improvement while also delivering concentrated skin nourishing and revitalizing ingredients.

Mechanism of Action

Nutrient rich fabric matrices maximize absorption potential using:

Occlusion - Creating a barrier prevents product loss into surroundings, allowing deeper penetration into stratum corneum reaching viable epidermal layers where collagen synthesis and pigment changes originate.

Time Release - Micro-encapsulation technology enables key ingredients like vitamin C, ceramides, peptides and antioxidants to gradually diffuse across dermal barriers over 30-90 minutes providing continual nourishment.

Compression - Adhesive pull from patches provides micro-compression smoothing fine lines while pressing bioactives into skin forcing diffusion across membrane improving efficacy.

Hydration Support - Hydrogels on back surface hydrate skin optimizing tissue permeability allowing better absorption unlike water loss prone creams. Dehydration impairs all rejuvenation.

Patches also provide ease of use allowing multitasking unlike more hands on creams or masks. Eye aesthetics improve cumulatively with committed use.

Considerations

When applying patch treatments:

Review Ingredients - Assess components first ensuring no personal allergens or irritants are included which may provoke puffiness or redness counterproductive to rejuvenating intent.

Follow Instructions - Adhere firmly to clean dry skin without overlapping for indicated 15-90 minutes based on encapsulated release profile. Resume normal skin care regimen after.

Use Sparingly - Limit eye patch use to three times weekly at most avoiding over reliance allowing skin recovery between treatments. Can dry out or provoke irritation with excessive use.

Specialized delivery masks and patches provide eye rejuvenating potential unmatched by standard topicals alone making them potent anti-aging allies in the battle against wrinkles, crepiness and darkening.

Makeup and Color Correctors

Skillfully applied makeup products provide immediate optical improvements minimizing the appearance of uneven pigmentation, dark circles, fine lines and puffiness. Color theory corrects shadows while light reflective particles impart plumping optics. Clever makeup application techniques transform eye aesthetics.

Correcting Discoloration

Strategic application of pigmented concealers and brighteners neutralizes dark hues using color theory:

Identify Undertone - Analyze skin color and circle darkness. Cool tones exhibit blue/purple hues. Warm tones appear more brown/orange. Select opposing hue.

Neutralize Shadow Color - Dab peach, orange or red-hued concealers on warm brown circles to counterbalance leaning into green color space. For blue-hued circles use yellow toned concealers which sit opposite on the color wheel.

Avoid Overbrightening - Don't apply excess brightener creating obvious reverse coloration or opaque caking. Sheer application balances natural skin luminosity.

With practice, corrective color selection adeptly obscures dark pigmented spots and blends naturally with surrounding skin for imperceptible amendments.

Diffusing Fine Lines

Softening the appearance of fine lines involving delicate tissues around the eyes leverages principles of light diffusion and distraction:

Primer - Smooth silicone primers over lids filling micro-crevices to create uniform surface minimizing shadows and flaws for light even distribution.

Luminizers - Dust slight shimmery highlights along upper orbital rims, cheekbones and inner eye corners drawing attention upwards with radiance. Distracts from lines.

Creamy Concealers - Hydrating, emollient concealers better fill in etched wrinkles unlike drying cakey formulas emphasizing cracks. Blend edges well.

Avoid Shimmers and Frosts - Reflective particles exaggerate crevices. Matte finishes hide shadows better through refraction of light at textural changes.

Makeup only provides optical trickery but clever application fosters eyes which distract from aging changes appearing flawless.

Minimizing Puffiness

Visual effects help deflate puffy eyes by contouring darkness and distracting with lines:

Cool Tones - Applying deep cool-toned concealer shadows along puffed lower lash lines pulls area inward for slimming effect.

Baking - Lightly press setting powder underneath eyes catching any oozing creams in texture camouflaging swelling.

Deflecting Lines - Draw upper and lower eyeliner arrows towards temples stretching eyes outward minimizing central puffiness.

Highlighting - Brighten inner corners and highlight brow bones with light shimmers drawing attention out and up away from puffy zones.

Like a magician redirecting attention, calculated color placement and optical illusions skillfully downplay tired swollen eyes.

Application Techniques

Finessing various specialized application techniques creates flawless eye enhancement:

Color Placement - After applying corrector and concealer use fingertips to gently tap and press into skin bonding pigments so movement and creasing doesn't lift coverage exposing darkness.

Blending Edges - Feather out concealer edges so no demarcation lines show. Blend down onto cheek skin so coverage fades seamlessly.

Baking - Lightly press setting powder under eyes and on lids setting concealers minimizing transfer and etched line emphasis. Let sit 30 seconds before dusting off excess with a fluffy brush.

Priming Lids - Smooth a sheer eyeshadow primer like a tinted base across lids providing uniform canvas allowing truer shadow colors and reducing creasing around fine orbital lines. Daily practice culminates in mastery allowing vision enhancement through illusion. Play with colors and lighting to redirect attention away from eye area flaws.

Redness Relievers

Irritation and dilation of surface capillaries surrounding eyes manifests as unsightly redness and inflammation distracting from one's sparkling gaze. Intermittently stressed eyes appear overtired. Soothing botanicals, anti-inflammatory peptides and green color correctors disguise red eyes.

Causes of Redness

Recognizing root causes guides solution selections to neutralize visible redness signature of irritation:

Allergens - Airborne allergens like pollen or dander provoke immune response releasing antibodies and pro-inflammatory histamines oozing fluid and blood byproducts into surrounding tissues appearing irritated.

Overwear of Contacts - Exceeding recommended contact lens wear time stresses corneal surface generating neurogenic inflammation and compensatory blood vessel dilation for oxygenation and healing.

Eyestrain & Fatigue - Prolonged intense focus strains ciliary muscles and dries surface tissues prompting reflex vasodilation response to nourish deprived cells giving bloodshot sclera appearance.

Injury & Surgery - Trauma from scratches, abrasions or injections permeabilizes vessels allowing blood leakage diffusely reddening eyes during healing phases.

Identifying the irritant or surface changes provoking redness allows mitigating response through lifestyle and topicals for visible improvement.

Soothing Botanical Extracts

Plant-derived anti-inflammatories relieve redness:

Aloe Vera - Mucilaginous gel coats and protects irritated ocular surface tissues and contains auxins and gibberellins which inhibit inflammation-propagating cytokines reducing redness signature.

Chamomile - Calming terpenoid chamazulene and flavonoid apigenin compounds decrease vascular permeability and prostaglandin-mediated inflammation giving red irritated eyes relief.

Green Tea - Epigallocatechin gallate (EGCG) inhibits collagen-chewing matrix metalloproteases and inflammation-signalling nuclear factor kappa B allowing inflamed eyes to heal faster with less blood vessel leakage reducing redness over time.

Peptide Complexes

Specialized peptides like palmitoyl oligopeptides and copper tripeptide target puffy eyes:

Palmitoyl Oligopeptide - Mimics collagen-stimulating growth factors prompting fibroblast activity for renewed dermal protein increasing tone and quickening healing.

Copper Tripeptide - Copper aids crosslinking of fibrous proteins like elastin and collagen while peptides signal tissue rebuilding communication cascades repairing damage faster with less irritation and redness.

Peptides accelerate repair so eyes appear less irritated faster while botanicals provide symptomatic relief and healing factors together reducing red, inflamed eyes.

Color Correcting Theory

Surface blood vessels reflect more red light waves accentuating appearance of diffusely red sclera and pink lids. Counterbalance with:

Primer - Smooth green-tinted primer over lids and orbits neutralizing resultant redness from irritated dilation. Green, as red's complementary color, conceals rosiness.

Conceal Red Areas - Spot conceal distinct vessels and pink patches after primer sets with fuller coverage yellow-toned concealer to balance redness. Yellow combats violet-blue hues blending seamlessly.

Skillful color correction obscures irritated ocular redness helping eyes appear fresh, rested and vibrant rather than overtired. Identify and avoid triggers while caring for delicate eye tissues.

Temporary Plumpers

Instantly restoring lost facial volume around eye areas prone to developing wrinkles and appearing hollowed revolves around effectively applying specialized primers, powders and contouring makeup. These props create optical illusions through distraction, refraction and shadows cultivating a refreshed and smoothed mien.

Primer Plumping

Optical primers containing light diffusing silicone polymers and microspheres instantly smooth over crevices and ridges to hide fine lines upon application:

Smoothes Skin - Silicones like dimethicone and cyclopentasiloxane fill micro-voids between skin cells and protein fibers creating a uniform surface scatter light more evenly hiding wrinkled texture and small folds around the eyes.

Contains Light Diffusers - Tiny uniform microspheres of nylon or silica bead primers refract incoming light waves hiding shadows of wrinkles. Rather than sink into crevices, light bounces creating youthful glow while obscuring hollowness.

Non-Comedogenic - Primers give the appearance of filled wrinkles without clogging pores which could worsen puffiness and skin health unlike comedogenic oils. Help keep eye area clear.

These special primers combine effective diffusion and filling properties instantly concealing fine eye lines when applied before other makeup.

Baking Shadow Effects

Strategic placement of matte setting powders adds contouring shadows visually receding areas seemingly fuller:

Under Eyes - Patting darker powder underneath eyes casts a subtle v-shaped shadow minimizing the look of bagginess and dark circles making region appear lifted without altering skin texture.

Outer Eyelids - Pressing deep tones along upper and lower lashlines in a connected v-shape along the outer eye corners creates illusion of receded eyelids making eyes appear wider awake.

Lower Lids - Dusting smoky-toned powder just below lower lashes makes eyes look larger by contrast since darker colors recede visually creating a more oval eye shape instantly.

Baking sculpted shadow effects distracts from tired appearance while optical makeup primers smooth away intricate crevices for rested eyes.

Volumetric Contouring

Custom shading mimics depth by strategic color placement:

Hollows & Circles - Dab oranges, peaches or yellows in hollows and circles then sheer and blend edges to balance darkness minimizing apparent dimension without lightening skin.

Eyelid Creases - Deepen natural upper eyelid crease indentations with neutral mid-range brown shadow which hides hooded appearance making eyes seem larger and more opened up.

Lower Lashlines - Add subtle definition along lower lash waterlines with closely matched brown or grey eyeliners which trace a slim shape without dragging eye downward visually.

Like a painter modulating light and shadows to create illusion of shape and depth, thoughtful makeup application sculpts beautiful eyes rediscovering youthful structure seemingly lost from repetitive strains of modern life.

Dark Circle Concealers

Stubborn dark pigmentation and shadows under the eyes draw attention away from brighter gaze. Thankfully specially formulated color correctors and concealers minimize darkened imperfections with light-manipulating pigments creating flawless coverage. Mastering these illusionist techniques transforms eye aesthetics.

Corrector and Concealer Differences

Specialized products address discoloration in targeted ways:
Color Correctors - Thickly pigmented creams with precise opposing undertones target neutralizing dark circle colors before standard concealing. Peach and red-orange correctors balance dark blue-purple circles. Green correctors counteract brown-red circles. Bright yellow camouflages surface redness and inflammation. Correctors are applied before concealer.
Concealers - Offer fuller coverage with skin matching hues to mask remaining darkness without adding ashen whiteness which can look obvious. Range of formulas in liquids, sticks and cakes seamlessly obscure residual discoloration, acne spots and flaws. Tap over correctors setting opacity.
Layering color correcting expertise under concealers ensures complete, natural coverage.

Ingredient Effects

Specialized ingredients within correctors and concealers create flawless eye transformation:

Light Diffusers - Ingredients like silica, mica and pearl pigments refract light waves hiding the shadows of dark circles rather than sunk within hollows giving brighter effect.
Soft Focus - Primers under concealers fill crepey fine lines making texture seem smoother so light scatters evenly instead of accenting cracks revealing concealed results last longer without gathering in folds.
Mechanical Fillers - Plumping spheres, nylon beads and hyaluronic acid temporarily expand tissue hiding vascularity

and thinness allowing better color coverage staying power. Help build creamy layer.

Innovative formulations truly hide imperfections instead of just covering darkly.

Application Techniques

Strategic application culminates in undetectable brightness:

Color Correct - Pat peachy corrector onto dark circles first counterbalancing tone before topping with concealer. Start with thin layer allowing gradual buildup to avoid unnatural paleness giving away makeup trickery.

Press into Skin - Instead of swiping or rubbing concealers onto delicate eye tissue possibly tugging and irritating, press and gently tap pigments encouraging absorption and bonding avoiding slipping into creases.

Edge Blending - Feather out concealer edges with fingertip so no distinct margin remains. Makeup fades more naturally blended into cheek skin for imperceptible application.

Masterfully applied concealers brighten entire eye aesthetics drawing sparkling forward from previous dullness or hollowness. Consistent technique creates flawless illusion every day.

Lash Enhancing Mascaras

Long luxurious lashes beautifully frame eyes making whites appear brighter, irises more vibrant and boosting lash line contrast. Special conditioning formulas increase lash volume, length and curl over time while tinting and thickeningeach fiber for immediate enhancement. Discover mascaras that magnify eyes daily.

Gradual Lash Improvement

Unique peptides and botanical extracts promote growth phases enhancing lashes with continued use:

Lash Lifting Peptides - Synthesized molecules like Myristoyl Pentapeptide-17, in which five amino acids link to a fatty acid, attach to hair follicles signaling growth factors biochemically prompting thicker healthier lashes to grow over weeks.

Botanical Growth Factors - Plant stem cells and extracts like those from clover flower andSwertia Japonica supply bioactive phytochemicals which nurture lash follicles improving output of keratin making lashes longer, more flexible and faster growing.

Lash Conditioning - Panthenol (Vitamin B5) and plant-based waxes coat lashes preventing brittleness and breakage while oils like argan penetrate softening lashes giving the appearance of thickness and length as more fibers remain intact.

Dedicated lash care mascaras boost follicle health revealing beautiful battable lashes.

Immediate Enhancing Effects

Specialized formulas optically enhance lashes immediately:

Carbon Black Pigments - Pure carbon molecules maximally absorb light creating intense black color unlike other muted pigments visually thickening lash fibers without clumping or flaking off. Makes lashes stand out boldly.

Microfibers & Nylon - Sparse or short lashes seem multiplied and lengthened instantly with tiny synthetic fibers interspersing between natural lashes adhering tint for boosted volume. Create fuller batting appearance immediately.

Lash Curlers - Manual or heated lash curlers shape lashes upwards opening eyes wider while also exposing lash lines more prominently especially useful for straight stubborn lashes.

Often incorporated with waterproof formulas preserving effects.

Clever cosmetic chemistry offers quick lash transformations while peptides and botanicals restore lackluster lashes long term.

Achieving Natural Enhancement

Balancing boldness with believability prevents clumpy artificiality:

Curl Base First - Begin mascara application using lash curler to lift lashes then coat bases with light handed pass of mascara before building color intensity on tips creating depth.

Wiggle Brush Application - Instead of gliding wand across lashes which can clump, gently wiggle bristles side-to-side separating and extending fibers preventing visible buildup.

Brush Separator Use - Alternate between applying product then using wand or separating comb specifically designed to redistributed clumped pigment for naturally enhanced individual strand separation.

Amplify eyes alluring windows by boosting lush lashes gradually or immediately without sacrifice. Discover multiplying mascaras that respect delicate lids nurturing enhanced growth and beauty over time.

Maintenance Routines

Consistent daily regimens cement cumulative benefits from targeted eye treatments over weeks and months preventing backsliding. Establishing maintenance habits protects improvements securing a perpetually refreshed eye appearance as we age. Dedicate just minutes twice daily.

Morning Routine

An invigorating morning routine enlivens eye appearance:

Cleansing - Remove residual night cream and accumulated tear film debris around eyes with a gentle pH balanced cleanser massaging outward from inner corners. Avoid soap irritation. Pat dry softly.

Massage - Invigorate circulation using light movements around the orbital bone from inner corners over eyelids outward above temples. Alternate tapping to move lymphatic fluids.

Serum - Treat topically with antioxidant Growth Factors and peptides which reinforce collagen structure around eyes helping sustain smooth skin. Tap serum gently around the contours without pulling.

Sun Protection - Shield thin eye skin from solar radiation and High energy visible light emitting electronics which degrade cellular integrity. Use broad spectrum SPF 30+ protection. Wear large lenses.

Morning maintenance solidifies rejuvenation gains keeping eyes looking well-rested and healthy consistently.

Evening Regimen

Nightly rituals renew eye revitalization:

Makeup Removal - Gently remove makeup, especially mascara and liners which migrate and irritate eyes overnight. Use bi-phase removers suitable for sensitive skin followed by rinsing.

Night Serum - Treat with specialized evening repair complexes containing Retinol, Bakuchiol or Alpha-Hydroxy Acids which resurface skin cells revealing brighter, less pigmented dermal layers overnight as we sleep.

Soothing Cream - Seal in serums with a rich night balm containing ceramides, peptides and hyaluronic acid to deeply hydrate delicate tissues from daytime environmental depletion.

Cool Therapies - Alternate chilled cucumber slices, rosewater spray mists and jade rolling to decompress eyes, improve circulation and lymphatic drainage minimizing accumulated daily burdens like fluid retention contributing to puffiness while supporting repair.

Consistent nurturing self care preserves hard won eye rejuvenation results maintaining your vibrant awakened eyes.

Seasonal & Situational Adjustments

We fine tune routines adapting to changing circumstances:

Altering Frequency - Use nourishing masks or intensive procedures less often in summer when skin is supple, and increase winter use combating parched air which dries eyes.

Managing Allergies - Supplement with oral antihistamines during high pollen seasons to control inflammatory reactions aggravating circles and puffiness. Rinse eyes post outdoor exposure.

Blue Light Filtering - Become more diligent minimizing digital device use and enabling screen filtering settings to protect eyes against oxidative high energy wavelengths when working longer hours or binge viewing.

Traveling - Pack separate contact lens cases, extra hydrating drops, firming eye gels, gentle cleansers and makeup removers conveniently accessible to properly care for eyes while journeying especially on planes which intensely dry eyes.

Customizing maintenance regimens preserves youthful eye revitalization results year round as situations shift through attentive care and protection.

Seasonal and Situational Plans

While essential daily routines preserve rejuvenated eyes, adjusting protocols to align with shifting seasonal environments and situational circumstances better sustains aesthetic progress. Customizing an eye care plan balances reactive treatment with preventative proactive modifications through the changing year.

Spring Plan

Blooming spring stirs joy but also seasonal allergy irritation for eyes:

Antihistamines – Surge in airborne pollen prompts immune hypersensitivity reactions release histamine causing puffy watery eyes. Take oral antihistamines daily throughout season to control response.

Hydration Boost - April showers and wind whip allergens drying delicate eye surfaces. Use thicker night creams around eyes and gentle rewetting drops to protect vulnerable cells from desiccation damage. Drink plenty of water.

Nutrition - Refresh diet with colorful berries and dark leafy greens to replenish antioxidants and anti-inflammatory bioflavonoids combating seasonal stress compounds attacking collagen integrity around the eyes leading to accelerated aging.

Welcome springs vital rebirth by honoring eyes sensitivity. Adjust protocols boosting hydration and circulation while controlling inflammatory pathways.

Summer Strategizing

Blazing summer sun and activities pose eye health hazards:
UV Protection - Shield eyes from burning rays with wide brimmed hats, properly chosen UV blocking contact lenses rated to filter radiation, and durable sunglasses worn regularly when outdoors preventing retinal damage and skin cancers around the lids.

Digital Device Limiting - Minimize seasonal surge in electronics use protecting eyes from oxidative high energy blue light emissions of phones, tablets and computers which generate free radicals degrading cellular integrity and draining visual stamina.

Travel Precautions - When journeying guard eyes against unfamiliar allergens and irritants by packing dedicated contact lens cases, hydrating gels, anti inflammatory rosewater sprays. Stay vigilant sourcing water quality maintaining healthy ocular surface.

Proactively preparing through summer safeguards vision while ensuring eye rejuvenation efforts continue uninterrupted by seasonal shifts. Adjust simplicity.

Autumn & Winter Strategizing

Crisp autumn's cozy appeal followed by harsh winter conditions intensely dry eyes necessitating added protection:
Hydrating Boosts - Heating, cold plunging temperatures and blustery conditions disrupt tear film lipid layers. Use thicker balms around eyes before bed supplementing with gentle hydrating gel drops upon waking to protect corneal surface cells. Consider humidifier at night.

Nutrition - Nourishing stews and roasted vegetables replenish depleted nutrient reserves from heightened summer activity ensuring adequate antioxidants protecting delicate eye vessels and muscles from seasonal cold stresses.

Blue Light Moderation - Limit electronic device use as days darken earlier reducing melatonin and straining eyes. Enable night shift screen settings. Soothing audiobooks or music provide calmer evening alternatives.

Guard against the elements through attentive seasonal shifts fine tuning eye supportive habits. Consistency carves the path towards sustained aesthetic eye rejuvenation for years.

Ongoing Eye Health Care

Maintaining eye health requires attentive self-care practices beyond aesthetic concerns to preserve vision and comfort. Routine eye exams, active monitoring, nutrition and eye hygiene sustain function allowing us to fully enjoy the vibrant appearance revitalizing treatments impart. Investing consistent efforts keeps eyes healthy for life.

Eye Exams

Seeing an optometrist or ophthalmologist routinely allows early detection of subtle changes impacting structure, fluids or optics before vision declines:

Comprehensive Evaluation - Exams check acuity, refractive errors, ocular alignment, focusing, coordination and depth perception to detect problems warranting correction like presbyopia or eye strain.

Eye Health Screening - Inspection inside the eye with dilation assesses internal changes like cataracts, retinal irregularities or optic nerve damage needing monitoring and secondary treatments to prevent complications like glaucoma or macular impacts.

Prescription Updating - As the lenses and shape of eyes shift slightly year-to-year, glasses or contacts prescriptions require periodic adjustment for best acuity matching internal changes maintaining sharp, comfortable vision.

Regular assessments safeguard precious sight and illuminate factors affecting overall eye vitality.

Self-Monitoring

Routinely self-checking specific parameters helps discern normal age-related changes from concerning pathology requiring medical care:

Clarity & Comfort - Note any difficulties reading, changes in light sensitivity or sensations of grittiness/irritation indicating surface dryness or refractive shifts which degrade visual functioning if not addressed.

Appearance - Inspect lids, lashes and white sclera with a magnifying mirror for symmetry, new vessels, pigmentation or suspicious lesions needing evaluation to rule out infection or skin conditions like blepharitis disrupting health.

Vision Function - Testing acuity daily with familiar text at usual reading distance checks ability to see fine details. Sudden onset blurriness, distorted images or obstruction warrant urgent assessment for retina/nerve disease. Being attentive allows rapid response to changes preventing major vision loss.

Protective Eyewear

Shielding eyes against environmental insults prevents surface irritation and deeper tissue damage:

UV Light - Exposure to ultraviolet radiation degrades sensitive ocular tissueMatrix increasing oxidative stress and cancer risk. Always wear 100% UV blocking sunglasses outside.

Foreign Bodies & Irritants - Safety eyewear creates essential barriers protecting delicate eyes from flying projectiles on job sites and wind-borne allergens irritating the surface. Side shields prevent particulate entry.

Digital Eyestrain - Filtering computer glasses reduce glare strain while selective light wavelength-blocking lenses ease focusing fatigue from intense blue light emitted by phones/screens. Alleviates dryness.

Safeguarding precious vision should motivate investing in durable, comfortable protective eyewear for all activities, work and play.

Eye Health Supplements

Key compounds in oral supplements demonstrate benefits combating common age-related vision changes:

Lutein & Zeaxanthin - These antioxidant carotenoids filter high energy blue light waves protecting retina cells from oxidative damage while improving glare recovery and contrast sensitivity declining with age.

Omega Fatty Acids - Daily fish, krill or algal oil capsules supply DHA shown clinically to improve dry eyes enhancing tear film stability and lubrication which commonly decline with age.

Vitamin C & E - These complementary antioxidants defend delicate eye tissues from free radicals generated through UV and blue light exposure from sun and screens sabotaging cells. Preserving structural integrity maintains function. Discuss adding these protective supplements with eye doctors to support ocular health long term.

Diligent self-checks, routine doctor visits, protective barriers and oral supplements sustain eyes for lifelong clear comfortable vision to fully enjoy rejuvenated aesthetics treatments impart. Prioritize total eye health with proactive care.

Committing to Your Vision

Having vibrant, youthful-looking eyes is about more than just aesthetics - it's about committing to a vision of health and vitality from the inside out. When we commit to proactive eye care, we are making an investment in our overall wellbeing for years to come.

Establish Daily Practices

The key to eye health maintenance is establishing simple, sustainable habits as part of your everyday self-care routine. Just 5-10 minutes a day focused on your eye area can make a significant difference over time. Some quick practices to start integrating:

 Gentle eye massages - use your ring fingers to apply light, sweeping pressure around the orbital bone. This stimulates blood flow and drainage.

 Hot and cold compresses - a warm washcloth followed by a cool jade roller opens up circulation.

 Soothing botanical tea bags - chilled green tea bags can instantly de-puff eyes.

 Targeted stretching - rotate your eyes clockwise and counter-clockwise. Look up, down, left, and right holding each gaze for a few seconds.

When these micro-practices become second nature, you are well on your way towards a lifetime of revitalized eyes.

Commit to Your Skincare Routine

Just like your daily eye wellness practices, be religious about your morning and evening skincare routines. The delicate eye area depends on regular nourishment and protection. Make products like these non-negotiable:

A dedicated eye cream - apply both morning and night. Look for formulas with peptides, vitamins C and E, and botanical oils.

Broad spectrum SPF - protect the vulnerable eye region from skin-aging UV damage. Mineral sunscreens are best for sensitive areas.

Nighttime repair treatments - creams with retinol or gentle retinoids renew the eye contour overnight.

Don't Forget the Basics

In our quest for bright, youthful eyes, we often overlook the simple foundational practices that make the biggest impact. No fancy product or high-tech procedure can replace core wellness basics like:

7-9 hours of sleep - quality rest is when tissue regeneration occurs. Sleep is a natural eye de-puffer!

A healthy, colorful diet - think leafy greens, carrots, tomatoes. Antioxidants nourish eyes from the inside out.

Hydration - water is essential for every bodily function, including healthy eyes and ease of drainage. Aim for at least 64 ounces per day.

Stress relief - anxiety and fatigue always show first in the delicate eye area in the form of wrinkling, dark circles and bags. Make relaxation a priority.

See Your Eye Doctor Regularly

While cosmetic eye care maintenance is worthwhile, it cannot substitute regular eye exams by your ophthalmologist or optometrist. They will screen for common age-related issues like:

Presbyopia - rigid eye lenses impact close vision

Cataracts - clouded lenses blocks light from entering the eye

Glaucoma - damage to the optic nerve

Macular degeneration - retina damage causes vision loss

Most conditions have few warning signs, making dilated eye exams critical. Catching problems early makes treatment more effective. Know your eye health baseline numbers and risk factors.

Address Changes Proactively

As you mature, be vigilant about subtle eye changes. Conditions like dryness and irritation, if left untreated, can spur inflammation and accelerated aging. Use these best practices:

Notice issues - stinging, redness, excessive watering all indicate potential eye trouble. Poor night vision or distance vision are other signs.

Identify triggers - from medication side effects to environmental allergens, pinpoint what provokes symptoms.

Seek solutions - treat dryness with ointments, avoid airborne irritants. See an optometrist for direction.

Don't assume eye changes are inevitable. There are always helpful interventions, both medical and natural.

Make Eye Longevity a Lifestyle

Rather than a quick fix, approaching eye rejuvenation as a lifelong endeavor is the smartest strategy. Support structures like collagen and elastin gradually decline with age. Regularly counteracting that breakdown can help eyes appear illuminated and lifted for decades longer.

Consistent gentle care protects the fragile periorbital skin against wrinkling and creping. Nourishing practices enhance anti-aging cell turnover too. Before expensive medical treatments are necessary, the small efforts make a cumulative difference.

Eyes are our window to the world. Protecting our sight and keeping eyes appearing fresh conveys vitality from the outside in. Vision clarity influences everything from safety to enjoyment of life's simple pleasures.

Prioritizing eye health maintenance ultimately invests in our independence and engagement with life. From hobbies like reading and arts to recognizing loved ones' faces, sharp eyesight enhances existence. Planning ahead allows us to see (quite literally!) the bright horizons ahead.

There is no better time than now to establish eye-focused directives. Consistent care and vigilance will pay rewards for years to come through brighter, firmer, more radiant eyes. Commit to your vision today!

Staying Consistent

Consistency is key when it comes to maintaining vibrant, youthful-looking eyes as you age. After putting in the work to find an eye care regimen that works for you, it's crucial to stick with it. Far too often, people start strong with a new routine only to slowly let it slide over time. They get busy or bored and stop doing all the little daily tasks that keep eyes looking refreshed and rejuvenated.

By buckling down and powering through when motivation wanes, you will reap the long-term eye and vision benefits from your savvy self-care rituals. This chapter will explore tips on how you can commit to consistency even when life inevitably throws roadblocks in your path.

Schedule Timeouts for Eye Care

Carve out designated times in your weekly calendar when you can properly focus your energy on eye rejuvenation tasks. For example, set aside 15 minutes each evening before bed when you'll have quiet alone time in the bathroom to apply eye creams, serums, gels, etc while enjoying some candlelight and soft music.

You might also schedule set times for eye exercises, soothing botanical compresses, gentle lymphatic drainage massages or other treatments that require concentration and thoughtfulness on your part. Even quick eye makeup removal and refreshing rinses warrant undivided attention.

By giving your eyes this sacred time, you are more likely to follow through day in and day out. The more consistent the love and care, the better your peepers will look and feel as the decades roll by.

Automate and Streamline When Possible

Find ways to seamlessly incorporate eye care into your daily routines so it becomes second nature rather than a chore. Maybe it's having jarred herbal tea compresses in the fridge ready to go each morning or keeping dark circle concealer right next to your toothbrush.

Prep pads and serums can live alongside your face wash and body lotion if that prompts you to swipe them on consistently. You can even set phone alerts reminding you to perform eye exercises or blink more frequently throughout the day.

When eye care duties meld with the rhythm of your lifestyle, you bypass excuses and encouraged to keep up the program. Consolidate, simplify and systemize.

Stick With A Core Regimen

While it can be tempting to sample every new eye innovation hitting the beauty aisles, it's best to stick with a simple, back-to-basics regimen for best results long-term. Find 5-6 core eye care products that work synergistically together and use them religiously before branching out and trying new "miracle" treatments.

Your regimen may include a nourishing overnight eye cream plus collagen-boosting serum in the mornings teamed with weekly botanical compresses and gentle lymphatic drainage massage. Or maybe you use a peptide complex morning and night along with hydrating hydrogel under eye patches.

Resist urge to constantly mix it up or else you won't really know what's working vs not. And your poor peepers will be confused by the constantly changing signals. Pick a handful of multitasking products that target your unique eye concerns then continue refilling them season after season.

Consider Subscriptions and Auto-Delivery

Running out of your must-have eye creams or serums can throw a major wrench in consistency plans. Consider signing up for auto-delivery subscriptions to ensure you never have a gap between shipments.

Many companies now offer monthly or bi-monthly shipping programs where you get your favorite products delivered straight to your door before running out. This eliminates frantic last minute runs to the store or stretches of time where you go without your regimen essentials. Auto-delivery helps guarantee consistency in using products long enough to accurately gauge results.

Team Up With Your Partner

Enlist your spouse or significant other to join you on your eye care journey. By applying creams, gels and serums together before bed or over morning coffee, you build in valuable accountability while making self-care routines more fun and bonding.

You can gently remind each other about eye exercises, screen breaks, herbals tea compresses etc if noticing one's consistency starting to slide week to week. Having your own personal eye care cheerleader helps incentivize sticking to all the little steps that maintain eye vitality decade over decade.

When persistent vision problems or severe dryness occurs that disrupt your regimen, consult an eye doctor for personalized guidance getting back on track promptly and safely. Sometimes minor procedures, prescription upgrades or ointments get you re-centered so you can continue progressing with your eye health goals.

Temporary hurdles and hiatuses will arise on any lifelong journey of optimal eye care. But by pre-committing to consistency no matter what, you give your eyes their best fighting chance to withstand aging's impact. With resilient determination and self-compassion during harder times, you will get back in rhythm again soon.

Eyes reveal so much inner beauty, creativity and wisdom. Commit now to caring consistently for your unique peepers so they continue conveying your spirit while light shines through clearly all along life's path.

Energy Levels and Eye Vitality

Our eyes are the windows to health and vitality - when we feel energized, our eyes appear more bright, refreshed and vibrant. But when energy tanks, our peepers pay the price. Fatigue shows in baggy lids, dark circles, dullness and lackluster lashes. Boosting overall stamina is key for revitalized eyes that dazzle. This chapter explores the close ties between whole body energy levels and eye health. You'll discover lifestyle tweaks that help fight fatigue so eyes appear well-rested and spirited at any age. Those telling tired eyes will perk right up when you implement an eye-friendly vitality plan.

Sleep and Eye Rejuvenation

Skimping on sleep is a surefire way to drain energy levels while accelerating visible aging in the thin delicate skin around eyes. Yet in our wired 24/7 world, fatigue is epidemic with the average adult getting just 6-7 hours sleep versus the 8-10 hours needed for optimal health and eye revival.

Prioritizing consistent high-quality sleep is perhaps the single best thing you can do for reducing eye wrinkles, puffiness, dark circles and lackluster eyes when you wake. While you rest, the body works diligently to heal cells, remove waste, consolidate memories, regulate hormones, restore energy and rally immunity.

Growth and anti-aging hormones like human growth hormone (HGH) peak while sleeping, working hard to repair cells and stimulate collagen production. Insufficient sleep throws this restorative work off track - you miss out on essential eye area rejuvenation leaving skin looking aged, eyes appearing tired.

Consistency is key for eye-enhancing sleep benefits so aim for the same bed and wake times daily, even on weekends. This stabilizes the body's circadian sleep-wake rhythms which cue reparative cellular activity over night. Develop a relaxing pre-bed routine that preps mind and body for sound slumber. Limit stimulating lights and digital screens in evening.

Dim lighting, eye masks, blackout curtains, white noise machines and cozy bedding all support quality sleep crucial for well-rested eyes. Don't underestimate power naps either - 10 to 20-minute daytime snoozes offer quick bursts of restorative energy that can brighten weary eyes in flash.

Nutrient-Dense Foods Energize Eyes

A vibrant diet rich in whole colorful fruits, vegetables, lean proteins, nuts/seeds and anti-inflammatory spices supplies necessary fuel for lively eyes. These nutrient-dense foods are high in antioxidants, phytochemicals and essential vitamins/minerals that nourish eyes and stoke sustainable energy stores.

For example, dark leafy greens like kale and spinach contain eye-healthy carotenoids lutein and zeaxanthin that filter blue light and quell inflammation. Bright orange produce bursting with betacarotene sharpens eyesight while deeply nourishing skin around eyes.

Wild caught salmon and grass-fed meats provide omega-3s that lubricate dry eyes, curb wrinkles and elevate mood. Complex whole grains like quinoa stabilize blood sugar for sustained stamina. And probiotic yogurt's good gut bacteria sparks whole body vitality, further powering bright beaming eyes.

So whip up an energizing breakfast hash with salmon, greens, eggs, avocado and berries. Lunch on a veggie quinoa bowl piled with chickpeas for sustained afternoon energy. Snack on nuts, seeds and hummus versus energy-sucking sweets which cause rebounds in blood sugar and fatigue.

Proper hydration is equally crucial so aim for 8-10 glasses of revitalizing liquids daily from pure water, green tea and the occasional coconut water for electrolytes. Liquids lubricate and brighten eyes while delivering nutrients blood and cells depend on for enduring, accessible energy to power dazzling eyes.

Exercise and Oxygenate Eyes

Regular exercise is a surefire ticket to boosted energy levels and peppy wide-awake eyes. Any moderate aerobic activity like walking, jogging, biking, dancing and swimming ramps up circulation delivering energizing, oxygen-rich blood throughout the body and to thirsty eye tissues.

Increased blood flow whisks away cellular waste buildup from eyes while transporting a steady supply of fuel, anti-aging and immunity boosting nutrients that recharge this delicate organ. Growth factors and proteins released during movement help strengthen eye structures and shore up protective barriers.

Aim for 30 minutes daily of cardio activity minimum to flood eye area with these revitalizing effects. Strength training's short bursts further oxygenate eye tissues for enhanced nourishment and vitality. And don't forget the lymphatic circulation benefits - having glam eyes means having healthy immune function and drainage which exercise supports.

Outdoor exercise offers extra perks for eye health - natural light triggers day-night circadian rhythms influencing hormonal cascades tied to energy levels and tissue regeneration. And spending time immersed in greenspaces gives eyes relaxing color therapy. Just be sure to wear UV-blocking sunglasses when outside to prevent damaging sun exposure.

Adaptogens Energize and Destress Eyes

For an extra eye stamina and aging defense boost, consider taking adaptogenic herbs like astragalus, ashwagandha, panax ginseng, rhodiola and holy basil in supplement form or as medicinal teas. These potent plant extracts help moderate cortisol stress hormones which can drain energy when chronically elevated.

By stabilizing adrenal and immune function, adaptogens build resilience to physical and emotional stressors that sap vitality and accelerate aging. This equanimity and fortitude directly supports eye health - balanced nervous system means rested relaxed eyes versus that telltale stress fatigue. The soothing, nourishing effects also bolster eye immunity and tissue repair capacity for lasting luminous peepers.

Relax and Recharge Weary Eyes

Make time each day to simply stop and let eyes relax - close them for 5-10 minutes while taking some deep cleansing breaths. Relax jaw, forehead and any frowning lines squinting up eyes. This short sensory timeout gives strained eyes and brain a break while triggering the relaxation response - a reverse shot of energy and circulation to weary eyes.

Use relaxing tricks like visualizing walking along a peaceful nature trail or laying on a warm sandy beach listening to crashing waves. Have eye drops handy to refresh any dryness or irritation as needed. Light an aroma therapeutic candle releasing calming lavender-pine scents. Simply stopping to honor eye health pays exponential energizing dividends long term.

Aim for vibrancy promoting behaviors and ample sensorial nourishment daily so eyes mirror back brilliance and vitality every time you catch their gaze. When energy, mood and immunity lag, vibrant eyes quickly fade turning lackluster. But revive whole body battery power through stellar sleep, active movement, wholesome dietary antioxidants and nervous system balancers and your eyes will dazzle with health regardless of phase of life. Make total body energy renewal a top priority and enjoy sparkling, magnetic eyes for decades to come.

Hormones and Puffy Eyes

Hormone fluctuations are a common culprit behind temporary eye puffiness, those annoying bags and swelling under eyes that can make you look tired, stressed or just plain old. As women we contend with monthly menstruation cycles plus perimenopause and menopause bringing roller coaster hormones that take eyes hostage.

Even men don't escape hormonal chaos as declining testosterone and insulin disruptions create headwinds. This chapter provides an overview of how reproductive, thyroid, growth and stress hormones impact eye health plus proven ways to smooth out their ruckus so you maintain gorgeous glowing eyes for life.

Estrogen and Eyes

Estrogen levels impact almost all tissues given receptors are found across body including delicate facial skin and collagen matrix around eyes. Estrogen supports healthy skin thickness, collagen production and elastin integrity for tautness. So the drastic drop during perimenopause and menopause leads to thinning dermis, slower cell turnover, declining structural proteins and fat redistribution.

Products penetrate eye tissue better with less subcutaneous fat too so irritants and allergens cause puffiness more easily. Estrogen is also vasoprotective helping blood vessels stay supple and oxygenated. Post-menopause vessel damage accumulates from oxidative stress. Weak parched vessels leak fluid into surrounding tissues causing inflammation and bags under eyes.

Estrogen therapy can help stabilize shifting levels while protecting eye blood flow. Discuss options with your doctor. Certain phytoestrogen botanicals like flax, red clover and maca may ease vasomotor symptoms too. Just take care with soy which can increase inflammation and stimulate tissue growth in those prone to fibroids or cancers.

Anti-inflammatory diet rich in cold water fish, greens, berries, tea and fermented foods helps temper symptoms too. Manage stress levels through yoga, meditation, breathwork, forests walks - this curbs cortisol which opposes estrogen compounding imbalance symptoms like eye puffiness. Consider probiotic supplements to support healthy gut flora which aids hormone metabolism and lymphatic drainage for reducing bags under eyes.

Progesterone and Eyes

Progesterone relaxes smooth muscle tissue causing vasodilation of blood vessels. Right before menstrual period when levels peak, eyes get puffy from leaky expanded vessels. Declining progesterone post-menopause allows vessel inflammation and oxidative damage to accumulate as aging progresses.

Without balancing estrogens, collagen synthesis declines and elastin fibers fray which show as creepy lines, wrinkles and eye hollowness. luckily the adaptogenic herb Chasteberry (Vitex) helps gently boost progesterone back to balance minimizing PMS symptoms like eye puffiness. Red Clover contains isoflavones that mimic estrogen and phytoprogesterone keeping vessels and skin around eyes supple.

Maca root is another medicinal herb that supports hormonal balance without overstimulating tissues. It modifies receptor site sensitivity helping maintain harmony as we age.Women battling monthly eye puffiness, bags and dark circles may ask doctor about continuous birth control pills which stabilize hormones. Discuss risks as synthetic hormones are not for everyone long-term.

Androgens/Testosterone and Eyes

Testosterone and its metabolites support healthy muscle tone and fat distribution in faces. Declines as men age leads to fat pockets, undereye hollowing. Testosterone strengthens skin collagen but less bioavailable versions from lowered output or conditions like high SHBG causes puffiness under eyes along with other visible aging signs.

Red light phototherapy boosts testosterone naturally by stimulating mitochondria while improving tissue oxygenation and lymph drainage. Limit stress and alcohol, lift weights, get adequate zinc/vitamin D to maintain optimal ratios. Saw palmetto and stinging nettle balance excess estrogen effects. But work with your doctor closely when supplementing with hormones male or female.

Thyroid Hormones

Thyroid hormones triiodothyronine (T3) and thyroxine (T4) regulate metabolism in every cell. Low thyroid slows cellular turnover, oxygen use, protein building, mitochondrial energy creation and waste clearance. Fatigue and exhaustion quickly show around eyes as dark circles and overt puffiness from pooled fluids and slower drainage.

Support thyroid function by minimizing stress, boosting nutrient density, removing gut irritants and strengthening digestion. Adaptogens like ashwagandha and seabuckthorn improve conversion of inactive T4 to active T3. Take care to get tested and work with your provider on proper treatment protocols if hypothyroid. Nourish thyroid and balance hormones for bright lively dazzling eyes!

Growth Hormone and Eyes

Growth hormone production declines steadily with age. By 60s it's a fraction of youthful levels. This negatively impacts body composition as muscle shrinks and fat accumulates especially around middle and face. Sagging skin, undereye bags result along with thinning eye collagen matrix causing hollows.

Boost natural growth hormones safely and sustainably through consistent strength training, high intensity interval training, adequate nightly sleep and smart supplement use. Consider collagen supplements with vitamin C plus radical scavenging antioxidants to defend youthful eye matrix as hormones shift.

Stress Hormones

Adrenaline, norepinephrine and especially cortisol release in response to stressful thoughts or situations. Short term this prepares us to fight flee or focus sharply. But modern times mean constant chronic stress pummeling body with excess stress hormones that break down collagen, clog lymph drainage, inflame tissues, stiffen vessel walls and impair immunity.

Results show fast around vulnerable thin eye skin - oxidative stress mottles skin with liver spots while weakening capillaries cause dark circles or visible spider veins. Puffy eyes happen as waste buildup overwhelms delicate drainage canals. Stress hormones frustrate other hormone pathways too stoking menopausal hot flashes or perpetual PMS. Mastering healthy stress responses empowers eyes to stay clear, calm and ageless regardless of life's pressures.

The takeaway? Supporting balanced endocrine function stabilizes biological rhythms for lasting eye health. Partner with your functional medicine doctor to identify imbalances early then gently guide hormones back to harmony through smart lifestyle tweaks, targeted nutraceuticals and routine screening labwork. Catching issues promptly preserves vibrant eye integrity decade after decade. Here's to ageless eyes and optimal endocrine health!

Gut Health and Eye Health

Ever heard the saying "the eyes are the window to the soul"? Turns out they are also a window into the health of our gut! The gut-eye axis is a very real mind-body connection. When gut balance is off, the eyes often signal distress quite visibly through symptoms like dark circles, redness, dryness and puffiness.

Supporting robust digestion and nurturing a flourishing microbiome lays a strong foundation for lasting eye health. So be sure to show your gastrointestinal system some love if you want clear, comfortable, ageless eyes! This chapter explains the gut and eye links then offers actionable steps for optimizing their symbiotic relationship.

The Gut-Eye Axis

The gut-eye axis encompasses the intricate immune and nervous system feedback loops connecting GI function with ocular health. Over 70% of immune system tissue resides in the digestive tract. Trillions of beneficial flora aid digestion, produce nutrients and metabolites and train immune cells.

A healthy flourishing microbiome keeps gut lining intact and immune function calibrated. Sensitive lymphoid eye tissue benefits through balanced immunoregulation and controlled inflammation. But when gut balance falters, chaotic immune signals can spark ocular inflammation.

Additionally tiny microvilli covering intestinal wall absorb nutrients from foods to nourish eyes and body. Dysbiosis and permeable leaky gut short circuit this nourishment pipeline. Poor absorption starves delicate eye structures. Deficiencies show as redness, cataracts, macular issues and compromised tear production.

The central nervous system links directly with enteric nervous system lining the digestive tract. This gut-brain axis sends signals in both directions affecting mood, stress responses, nerve signals to organs, pain perception and more. ENS irritation from bad flora, toxins or food reactions generate neuro-immune signals that strain eyes.

Signs of Eye Distress From GI Imbalance

How do you know if your eyes are trying to signal gut troubles? Be on the lookout for these common manifestations:

- Frequent styes
- Blepharitis (eyelid inflammation)
- Meibomian gland dysfunction
- Dry, gritty eyes
- Dark under eye circles
- Puffy eyes
- Bloodshot whites
- Light sensitivity
- Blurry vision
- Eye twitching

Sudden onset of symptoms like redness, swelling and ocular pain may indicate gut infection from bacteria or parasites. Seek medical care promptly in such cases. More insidious chronic low gradedigestive imbalance creates gradual changes in eye comfort and appearance. Tackle root causes before permanent damage sets in.

Healing the Gut-Eye Axis

Want to show your peepers some gut-healing love? Here are some top ways to realign this vital axis:

Remove Irritants and Toxins

Eliminate notoriously hard-to-digest foods like gluten, dairy, corn, soy and factory farmed eggs and meats. Toxins from mold, heavy metals, plastics and cosmetic chemicals burden detox organs compromising elimination. Avoid GMO foods too - glyphosate residues damage gut lining. Give digestion a fresh start by clearing out anything provocative.

Test for Pathogens

Do you suspect gut infection - whether bacterial, viral or parasitic? Explore specialty stool, blood or breath tests to identify the root organism(s). Stop guessing and treat the true offender for lasting relief. Culturing good guys alongside eliminating bad bugs rebalances terrain.

Prioritize Prebiotic Plant Foods

Prebiotics are the non-digestible fibers and resistant starches that feed healthy flora so they flourish. Load up on garlic, onion, leeks, asparagus, Jerusalem artichokes, sweet potatoes, yams, yucca root, dandelion greens, seaweed and apples. The broader the variety the better to nourish diverse microbes.

Consume Fermented Probiotic Foods

Sauerkraut, kimchi, beet kvass, coconut kefir, kombucha, miso, tempeh and yogurt offer complementary nourishing probiotics. Mix into meals regularly to maintain microbial diversity and ideal ratios of strains. This restores equilibrium between good guys and troublemakers. Avoid added sugars which feed disruptive yeasts and fungi.

Strategically Supplement Probiotics

Look for potent broad spectrum probiotic blends with at least 30 billion CFUs from reputable brands. Prioritize ones containing Saccharomyces strains which shape eye health. Pair with prebiotics for optimal nourishment results. Rotate through different targeted products seasonally meeting needs of ever changing inner ecosystem.

Soothe With Slippery Elm or Marshmallow Root

The mucilaginous herb slippery elm coats, protects and soothes irritated gut lining allowing regeneration of tight junctions sealing the barrier against future insults. Similarly marshmallow root gel heals ulcerations that permit particles accessing bloodstream triggering eye reactions. Sip as healing teas or take supplements.

Balance Blood Sugar

Excess blood glucose feeds yeasts like candida that damage gut integrity. Meanwhile vascular tissue throughout the body stiffens from glycation speeding aging. Tightly control carbs while emphasizing anti-glycative foods like carnosine-rich poultry, berries and brightly pigmented produce. Metformin may help moderate glucose swings too.

When the gut stays happy, eye health reaps rewards through balanced immunity, efficient nourishment channels and minimized inflammation. Support healthy digestion with prebiotic and probiotic bounty while eliminating irritants. This relieves strain on the gut-eye axis so peepers stay clear and comfortable reflecting soulful vitality.

Whole Body and Eye Circulation

Robust circulation is the fountain of youth for vibrant eyes at any age. Nutrient-rich blood transports oxygen, antioxidants, phytonutrients, proteins and moisture to thirsty eye structures while whisking away metabolic waste. Sluggish circulation fails to adequately nourish or detoxify, accelerating visible aging.

Supporting healthy blood flow holistically pays dividends through brighter sclera, reduced dark circles, faded spider veins and eye skin that stays plump and hydrated. Read on for lifestyle tips boosting circulation from head to toe for lasting bright-eyed vitality.

Exercise and Eye Blood Flow

Make daily movement a priority for keeping blood pumping strongly to eyes. As little as 30 minutes of moderate cardio activity sends oxygenated blood circulating while strengthening vessel walls. Even light walking helps. Just avoid straining which increases internal pressure.

Focus on relaxing, fluid movements like gentle swimming, cycling, dancing, yoga and tai chi. Strength training boosts blood vessel development too. And don't forget the value of deep cleansing breaths - inhaling fully oxygenates blood then full exhales dispel waste-laden air.

Inverted postures like downward dog, headstands and shoulder stands leverage gravity helping blood drain from eyes so vessels rest. This reduces pressure and strain. But avoid poses that spike blood pressure behind the eyes like handstands.

Massage Supports Eye Circulation

Massage boosts blood and lymph flow which nourishes and detoxifies eye tissues. Using gentle pressure, massage across eyebrows, along nasal bone and under eyes moving outward toward ears. This follows lymphatic drainage pathways. Repeat a few times daily.

Cool jade and rose quartz facial rollers feel soothing during this massage ritual. Or treat yourself to regular professional face and eye massages for a more thorough circulation surge. Just be sure therapists use gentle pressure and proper technique around delicate eye blood vessels.

Manage Blood Pressure

Uncontrolled hypertension strains the tiny vasculature nourishing the eyes due to excess pressure. Over time this causes microtears and weakness leading to fluid leaks, macular damage and vision changes. Keep blood pressure ideally below 120/80 through diet, exercise, stress relief and medication if necessary.

Emphasize heart-healthy foods like wild-caught fish, nuts, olive oil, oats, beans, non-starchy veggies and berries in anti-inflammatory patterns like Mediterranean diet. Limit sodium and saturated fats. Stay lean and active to take advantage of exercise's BP-lowering, vessel-protective effects. Address stress through yoga, mindfulness, nature immersion and social connection. Consider supplements like aged garlic, hawthorn berry, cocoa flavanols and coenzyme Q10 too.

Balance Blood Sugar

Excess blood glucose from poor carbohydrate metabolism glycates and inflames vascular structures everywhere accelerating aging. Keep blood sugar stable through smart meal spacing, carb portions and pairings that prevent spikes and crashes. Emphasize high fiber whole foods, protein at each meal and cinnamon which helps shuttle glucose out of circulation into cells.

Clean up diet by removing pro-inflammatory refined grains, factory farm meat/dairy and fried/packaged snacks. Up vegetable content and increase healthy fats while moderating total carb portions. Consider adding a gluco-balancing nutraceutical like berberine, bitter melon or ALA. Upping exercise helps reverse insulin resistance too.

Target Eye Antioxidants

Antioxidants protect delicate eye blood vessels and nerves against free radical damage from UV exposure, smoke and other pollution. Boost intake of vitamins C and E plus plant pigments lutein, zeaxanthin and astaxanthin. These neutralize oxidative stress preserving vascular integrity so eyes stay nourished and waste-free.

Bilberries and other dark berries offer bioflavonoids that strengthen capillaries stopping leaks while improving blood flow. The omega-3 DHA fortifies vessels too. Consider an eye health supplement with this antioxidant, anti-inflammatory combo for all-in-one insurance against aging. Just run additions by your doctor first with any medications.

Alternate Hot & Cold Compresses

Soothing hot and cold compresses around the eyes stimulate circulation in the veins and lymph. The alternating temperatures constrict then dilate vessels tricking them into pumping fresh nutrient-rich blood through while removing waste buildup. This reduces blood stagnation and puffiness.

Use a soft clean washcloth soaked in warm water for 30 seconds then switch to cool water for another 30 seconds. Repeat cycle 5-10 times 1-2 times daily for refreshed, nourished eye area circulation. Discontinue if irritation results and avoid extreme temperatures to prevent burns.

Dry Brush Skin Toward Heart

Invigorating whole body dry skin brushing performed toward the heart reactivates stagnant surface blood and lymph drainage which revitalizes eyes. Using a soft natural bristle brush, start at feet brushing upward in long strokes on front and back of legs before moving up torso and arms. Finish with neck and chest.

Aim for 5-10 minutes daily prior to showering so impurities dispel down the drain. Skin emerges softer, circulation stimulated carrying nutrients and oxygen out to eye tissues through healthier vessels while uprooting toxins. This holistic ritual leaves eyes brighter within weeks.

When you nourish a healthy head-to-toe circulation system through diet, movement and self-care practices eyes reap rewards. Adequate blood flow prevents waste accumulation while delivering essential anti-aging, antioxidant and hydrating elements. Commit now to lifelong circulation support for resilient clear eyes.

Managing Blood Sugar

Balancing blood sugar is a pivotal piece of the eye health puzzle at any age. When glucose metabolism works efficiently, the eyes thrive on a steady supply of this crucial energy molecule. But uncontrolled swings in sugar from poor diet or lifestyle habits spell disaster for eye tissues.

Excess blood glucose and its downstream effects like inflammation, glycation damage and sluggish circulation accelerate aging in delicate eye structures. Read on to understand how managing glucose intelligently preserves eyes that dazzle decade after decade.

How Blood Sugar Impacts Eyes

Glucose is the essential fuel cells depend on to create energy and power bodily functions. After consuming carbohydrates, the digestive process breaks these molecules down into various sugars including glucose which enters the bloodstream.

The pancreas releases insulin allowing glucose shuttle from blood into cells. When circulating glucose gets too high, excess sticks to proteins and lipids throughout body via glycation forming sticky inflexible AGEs (advanced glycation end products). This causes tissue stiffness, damage and accelerated aging.

Eyes are especially vulnerable as the thin skin contains minimal structural proteins like collagen to begin with. When what little matrix exists becomes overwhelmed by AGEs, noticeable wrinkling around eyes develops fast. Extreme vascular permeability means sugars inside blood seep out damaging surrounding nerves and muscle.

Fluctuating blood sugar also strongly influences fluid balance. Excess glucose pulls water into vascular spaces causing puffy eyes while rapid drops later pulls liquid away draining eyes. These ongoing shifts fatigue supportive muscles and ligaments leading to sagging eyelids over time.

Controlling Carb Intake

The quantity and quality of carbohydrates consumed directly impacts how efficiently the body processes and utilizes blood glucose. Refined grains, starchy vegetables and sugary treats spike sugar too fast for cells to keep up with leading to systemic buildup and overflow into tissues.

Focus carbohydrate intake instead around low glycemic options like non-starchy veggies, beans/legumes, nuts, seeds and 100% whole intact grains. The fiber, protein and fat naturally present helps slow digestion preventing rapid glucose spikes. Spread smaller carb portions throughout day rather than concentrating at any one meal for steadier energy.

Limit obviously sweet treats plus even unassuming culprits like commercial bread, crackers, cereals, sauces and dressings which concentrate refined carbs. Always pair carbs with fiber, protein and health fats to buffer blood sugar response. For example oatmeal with nuts and berries stabilizes better than a packaged muffin.

Portion control is key for those struggling with blood sugar imbalance issues. Work with a nutritionist or functional doctor to define ideal grams of carbs per meal and intake timing. This helps retrain body's glucose handling over time through consistent blood sugar stability.

Incorporate Blood Sugar Balancing Foods

Certain superfoods contain compounds that directly blunt glucose spikes and enhance cell insulin receptivity for optimum sugar utilization. Incorporating these regularly buffers sugar swings promoting eye health:

Cinnamon - Potent antioxidant and anti-inflammatory spices that mimics insulin shuttling glucose into cells

Berries - Rich source of anti-glycative anthocyanins

Green tea - Catechin EGCG reduces insulin resistance

Apple cider vinegar - Acetic acid slows digestion lowering glycemic response

Fatty fish - Omega-3s reduce inflammation enabling better insulin function

Chia seeds - Glucose regulating alpha-linoleic acid (ALA)

Emphasizing anti-inflammatory foods like leafy greens, deeply hued vegetables, omega-3-rich seafood, nuts, seeds and antioxidant spices further helps mitigate downstream effects of surplus glucose like vessel damage and tissue breakdown.

Exercise and Blood Sugar

Inactivity allows blood glucose to stagnate and concentrate rather than effectively entering cells to power activity. Just 30 minutes daily of moderate cardio exercise like walking vastly improves insulin receptor sensitivity and glucose clearance from blood.

Strength training offers similar balancing effects - working muscles eagerly gobble sugar from circulation. The body becomes more adept utilizing and storing glucose rather than letting excess accumulate triggering tissue damage. Moving daily provides compound eye benefits by stabilizing blood sugar, enhancing circulation and detoxification, pumping nutrients in and flushing wastes out.

Targeted Nutraceuticals

Certain botanicals and nutritional compounds directly improve glucose metabolism, insulin function and glycation processes benefitting eye health:

Chromium - This trace mineral boosts cell receptivity to insulin for better sugar uptake

Berberine - Alkaloid from goldenseal and Oregon grape helps lower unhealthy visceral fat that drives insulin resistance

Bitter melon - This tropical vine fruit controls excess hepatic glucose production by the liver decreasing output

ALA - Alpha lipoic acid mimics insulin escorting glucose from blood into cells

Resveratrol - Potent red grapes antioxidant activates the SIRT1 longevity gene improving mitochondrial energy creation from glucose

Magnesium - Critical cofactor for over 300 enzymes including glucose metabolism reactions

Research optimal doses for your needs and discuss combos with your functional doctor. Thing botanicals and vitamins amp up standard diabetes medications so adjustments likely needed if mixing. Get guidance adjusting quantities safely.

Stress Less For Balanced Blood Sugar

Chronic stress overactivates the fight or flight nervous system causing excess stress hormone release like cortisol and norepinephrine. These messily trigger blood sugar spikes and crashes which strain the pancreas' insulin output trying to perpetual catch up.

Make time to actively relax through yoga stretches, meditative breathing, forest walks and other calming rituals that engage the parasympathetic nervous system. This signals the body to downregulate stress systems providing a reprieve to regulate blood sugar more smoothly. Consider adaptogens like rhodiola and ashwagandha to calm excess cortisol release too.

Balancing blood sugar intelligently minimizes glycosylation damage of eye tissues while providing steady accessible fuel for cells. Be proactive against metabolic dysfunction and loss of insulin sensitivity early on for lasting eye health through middle age and beyond. Vibrant eyes reflect inner harmony!

Self-Care and Self-Love

Caring for your eyes is, at its core, an act of self-love. It demonstrates respect for your body and a commitment to your health and wellbeing. However, in our busy modern lives, self-care often falls by the wayside. This chapter explores how to cultivate self-love through a lens of nurturing eye health practices. You'll discover how slowing down to care for your eyes is a beautiful act of self-compassion with ripple effects across your whole being.

Carve Out Sacred Self-Care Time

In our distracted digital age, it's essential to consciously carve out tech-free space for self-nourishment. Rather than squeezing in quick eye cream applications while multitasking, set the intention to wholly devote relaxed quality time to eye care rituals.

Dim the lights, put on soothing music, and clear away clutter around your space. Sit comfortably and take a few deep cleansing breaths while gently massaging eyes. Apply serums, gels and masks with full presence while visualizing revitalization.

Use the time to practice mindfulness, consciously releasing any tension around eyes and forehead. Feel the skin absorb nourishing ingredients while eyelids grow heavy, inviting rest. These quiet mini-retreats renew spirit while refreshing eyes. Schedule them into each day like any other important commitment.

Disconnect From Digital Overload

In recent decades, screen time has exploded - televisions, computers, smartphones exposing our eyes to endless artificial light and sensory stimulation. This overwhelms delicate nerves and structures leading to strained tired eyes accompanied by attention challenges, headaches, insomnia and even emotional distress.

Set reasonable limits on recreational screen use to prevent burnout. Notice how eyes feel after scrolling social media or binging shows - sensitivity, fatigue and discomfort signals overload. Carefully close devices giving eyes candle-lit tech-free restoration offline. Long term limiting digital input preserves vibrancy while strengthening attention spans.

Journal About Self-Care Insights

Reflect on when you feel most nourished and which actions deplete energy. What self-care brings joy versus duty-bound exhaustion? Track experiences in a journal to identify optimal balancing rituals for eye and life vitality.

Color code entries by categories like nutrition, hydration, sleep, supplements, treatments, socializing, nature immersion, recreation etc. Note associated moods and eye comfort Too. Patterns reveal ideal regimens and doses of each area. Refer back when designing personalized plans.

Surround Yourself With Inspiration

Use imagery and affirmations that inspire eye care commitment. Post photos of yourself with vibrant shining eyes as a reminder of your potential. Cut out magazine pictures representing self-love goals like confident women with radiant skin or couples laughing over vegetables.

Write positive mantras on mirrors like "I nourish my eyes with love" and "My eyes sparkle with spirit". Let these become touch points focusing intention on uplifting actions. Shift environment to continually reflect self-care priorities back.

Indulge Other Senses Too

While vision is critical, don't overlook other senses equally deserving TLC for whole being balance. Savor tasty nutritious home cooked meals, massage tired feet with essential oils and soak them in lavender Epsom salts. Luxuriate in steaming aromatherapy showers, spritz on refreshing orange flower water mist.

Surround yourself with tactile softness - silk robes, velvet pillows, soothing eye masks and thick cozy socks nurture touch-starved skin. Bring beauty to all five senses through flowers, candles, music and potpourri. Fulfilling sensory needs breeds emotional satiation that ripples out to eye glow too.

Ask For Support From Loved Ones

Caring for your eyes better doesn't mean going it alone. Share goals with loved ones who can hold you accountable on tougher days. Have them remind you about screen breaks, sunglasses and session eye massages when willpower lags. And in turn offer reciprocal help with their health objectives.

Plan creative incentives like cooking nutrient dense dinners together or enjoying a girls spa night doing DIY facials. Send encouraging texts checking on regimen consistency. Cheer each other on through inevitable ups and downs. Shared commitment breeds collective momentum that lifts all spirits.

True self-care stems from a deep belief you are worthy of love, attention and nurturance. It means honoring feelings, thoughts and bodily needs rather than suppressing them. Extend this compassion towards your eyes too - make time to refresh and fortify them as an act of whole being adoration. When you lead with self-love, confident eye vitality naturally follows.

Aging Gracefully

Aging brings natural changes to our eye anatomy and function. But by embracing this evolution gracefully, we allow our inner light to shine brighter even as time marches onward. This chapter explores how to make peace with the aging process through spiritual principles and holistic practices that support eye health in alignment with your stage of life.

You'll discover timeless wisdom for vital eyes regardless of age while learning to see beauty in every phase of the lifelong journey.

Accepting Impermanence

Coming to terms with the ephemeral nature of life is the heart of aging gracefully. All phenomena - our bodies, thoughts, relationships and possessions - exist only transiently. Nothing in the material world is permanent.

Yet we suffer trying to cling to health, beauty, titles, accomplishments - attaching identity and worth to these changeable things. When youth fades, it feels like loss of self. But turning attention instead to life's inevitable ebbs and flows alleviates suffering.

Develop equanimity through spiritual practices like meditation, yoga, prayer or nature immersion. These reveal that beyond the physical world lies timeless universal consciousness welcoming us always like the ocean cradling waves. You are and always will be far more than mere eye bags or wrinkles.

Focusing on Gratitude

Life offers endless gifts if we pause to notice them with gratitude. The mere ability to see at all is precious. Honor eyesight by fully engaging its magic - watching sunsets, getting lost in art, beholding loved one's faces.

Catalog in a journal the sights, scents, textures and sounds that bring joy and meaning. Refer back when struggling so little daily miracles override aging's trials. Write thank you notes to your eyes for decades of colorful vistas. Feel blessings wash discomforts away.

Broadening Perspective

Consider the totality of your lived experience - challenges overcome, wisdom gained, adventures spanning the gamut of emotions. Appreciate all who crossed your path teaching about humanity. Distill lessons that now offer guidance to others.

This life view stretches far beyond surface-level aging concerns, putting changes in perspective. We dwell too narrowly on sagging skin when soul spans infinity. Regularly practice expansive thinking via meditation, psychotherapy, creativity, prayer or philosophical debate.

Connecting with Community

Find common ground with those in other seasons of life through heart-centered communication. Share respective struggles and triumphs. Recall how fleeting youth once felt despite yearning for those bygone days now.

Through community bonds we transcend fixation on wrinkles and impaired vision, instead reaching mutual understanding. You may inspire younger generations while a teen's innocence captivates your inner child once more. We age together, all on same path at different mile markers.

Nourishing Inner Light

External youth fades allowing inner radiance to beam brighter without competition - like stars coming out at dusk. What soulful gifts waiting to be shared once ego steps aside? Consider late stage life purpose - teaching universal truths, volunteering, creating artworks imbued with profound compassion.

Your inherited wisdom now ripens if given space through spiritual nourishment practices like chanting, dream journaling, divinatory rituals (Tarot, I-Ching). Shedding false beliefs about fading value frees you to shine.

Caring Holistically at Every Age

Diligently support eye health needs matching current phase. Childhood requires careful UV protection, nutritious diet and strong reading glasses if needed. Regular screen breaks preserve sight still developing.

Come young adulthood, begin preventative care. Antioxidants defend against damage while collagen-boosting peptides and retinoids build structural matrix protecting for later years. Protect vision with routine eye exams.

From peri-menopause forward monitor changing hormonal influences like dryness while promptly addressing new floaters, vision changes or eye discomfort indicating disease. Supplement tear production, attend to related health factors like blood pressure/sugar control and maximize nutrition fighting oxidative stress.

Respond swiftly if problems arise like cataracts or glaucoma; many cumulative vision issues become irreversible if left unchecked. Support aging eyes proactively yet gently. They crystallize life's beautiful impermanence.

Aging's superficial losses peel back pure consciousness to revel who you've always been beneath - eternal, boundless, radiant spirit. Anchor here as body naturally evolves, at peace with lovingly maintained eyes mapping lifetime's travels.

True Beauty Comes From Within

Eyes may be windows to the soul, but inner radiance and self-acceptance ultimately determine their magnetism regardless of flawless anatomy or unwrinkled texture. Lasting eye beauty stems from spiritual qualities like compassion, gratitude and equanimity rather than superficial traits we fixate on.

This chapter explores how befriending perceived imperfections then nurturing innate gifts allows unique inner light to channel through eyes, attracting others through authentic presence versus temporary arrangements of collagen and pigments.

Discover how to know, heal and freely express your whole being for confident eyes sparkling with spirit from within.

Observe Judgmental Thoughts

Notice judgments arising about your eyes' appearance - too small, uneven, puffy etc. Write these criticisms down without analysis. Recognize this harsh self-talk as conditioning, not truth. Our culture fixates on static plastic standards ignoring inner strengths defining authentic beauty.

Now imagine gazing into a loved one's eyes seeing past shape, hue or wrinkles. How do warmth, wisdom, wit glimmer through despite aging changes? Recall times eyes touched your soul.

Could anyone critique ears for not matching perfectly? Or hair for thinning over time? Eyes equally deserve loving patience not demanded mechanical perfection. Start simply witnessing judgments detached. Then consciously release those thoughts on exhale while thanking eyes for their faithful service.

Honor Eye Uniqueness

Consider the improbable factors that created your iris coloring, size, spacing and shape. Beginning as embryonic stem cells, proteins drove eye formation in utero per encoded DNA inherited randomly combining parents' eye elements from their conception.

Billions could have manifested. But only these eyes came to be - utterly rare jewels in history of human existence. Even genetically identical twins show subtle iris variation. That makes your eyes miraculous works of ephemeral art. Thank them for gracing planet.

List special attributes - alluring speckles dotting one iris, an endearing prominent fold, or distinctive limbal ring gracing the edge. Fall in love with exactly how eyes show up frame after frame. This is the vehicle spirit chose. So honor that!

Grow Self-Acceptance

Radical self-acceptance requires relinquishing any lingering eye shame stemming from perceptions you don't measure up. Who handed down those narrow beauty constructs anyway?

Certainly not the divine inner light recognizing all incarnating souls as equals.

Try gazing at eyes in mirror while saying positive mantras like "My eyes are perfect for me." "I lovingly accept my eyes." "My eyes show my soul." How does energy shift meeting their gaze? Keep reflecting inward until shame dissolves, embedding self-compassion as permanent mental overlay.

Live Eyelid Affirmations

Combat conditioned beliefs that eyes must look a certain youthful way by posting little affirmations actually on eyelids! Using non-toxic gentle adhesive strips made for eyes, apply tiny messages stating "I shine at every age!" or "Wisdom grows within". Read them to yourself while blinking throughout day. Silly? Perhaps. But so are society's restrictive signposts demarcating when eyes presumably gain or lose beauty based on age. Condition conscious and subconscious minds through positive eyelid affirmations! Then watch outmoded assumptions about eye value based on temporary looks start fading fast.

Express Your Authentic Self

Instead of camouflaging perceived eye flaws trying to meet unrealistic beauty ideals, courageously emphasize what makes you uniquely you. Play up distinctly hooded lids with smoky lavender shadow or leopard spots with bold graphic liner. Show the world exactly what beauty lives here through unapologetic self-expression.

Spend time connecting to abiding soul presence under temporary aging issues layered atop eyes. What untamed creative force yearns to shine regardless of shapes and sizes? Unleash your distinctive wild rainbow spectrum through eyes without worrying over perfect presentation.

Relax The Gaze

Much eye tension and squinting attempting to control outward appearances actually suppresses our lively spirit. Constant image management is exhausting! Train eyes instead to relax into natural form through deep exhalations while focusing gaze gently inward or at middle distance.

Soften eyelids, smooth brow furrows and release grimace lines by consciously relaxing face muscles multiple times daily. Shake off judgment whenever catching reflexive glances into mirrors or phone cameras too. Reprogram untamed eyes to live freely not fearfully monitored. Inner light beams brighter through relaxed eyes.

As physical beauty naturally evolves over decades, consider pivoting focus to unfolding spiritual gifts long muted by emphasis on appearances - compassion for humanity's shared struggles, equanimity in the face of conflicting desires, wisdom to uphold dignity and grace through life's losses.

Such soul strengths reign eternally making transient wrinkles seem trivial by comparison. Commit to uplifting inner luminosity and watch outer sparkle through eyes become merely side effect. True beauty needs no mirrors. Honor what inherently shines inside already complete and ageless.

Confidence Cultivation

Self-assurance stems not from meeting rigid external constructs of eye beauty but rather from bold embodiment no matter what eyes show up. By bravely being our authentic selves including embracing changing traits like wrinkles or age spots, we exude magnetic confidence that cannot be mimicked through makeup alone. This chapter explores building real eye confidence through spiritual principles, mental practices and holistic self-care rituals. Discover how to shine regardless of temporary surface-level eye qualities!

Connect with Inner Wisdom

Close eyes. Breathe deeply while scanning senses - muscles relaxing, sounds fading as thoughts drift by like clouds. Keep sinking further inward until reaching vast glowing inner sanctum, your core essence beyond transient aging or appearances.

Abide here fully embraced by eternal presence. Then bring bare awareness back up through body on next inhale, noticing eye chambers last. Hold compassion for these portals before softly re-opening the lids. After practicing this often, inner wisdom overlay sticks, trumping external cues attacking self-worth. Confidence blooms from within.

Neutralize Critical Self-Talk

Notice judgments arising about eye crinkles, dark circles, unevenness etc. Write down critiques without analysis. Now list 3 objective compliments about eye function despite disliked traits - perhaps beautiful iris colors, emotive expressions or reliable coordination still with vision.

Thank eyes for working so hard to bring you sights, smiles and intimate bonds. Conclude by writing a balanced affirmation like "My eyes show appropriate signs of joyful living and serve me well overall". File paper away as record of thought reconditioning.

Celebrate Eye Character

Wabi-sabi is the Japanese art of appreciating beauty in things imperfect, temporary and incomplete - like the cherry blossom's fleeting bloom or crackled glaze on ancient pottery. Apply this mindset to eyes. Consider each fine line crowding lids not bothersome defect but rather proud marker of smiles lived fully.

View mottled eyelid skin as Watercolor canvas conveying whimsical life narratives. Can you decipher stories inked into that tapestry etched by cycles of worry then optimism, heartbreaks and triumphs? Squint happily knowing eyes locked into your past and now too.

Focus On Self-Improvement

The most confident individuals concentrate not on anxiously analyzing perceived flaws but rather staying focused improving current skills while developing new ones. They know our worth comes from courageously sharing personal talents versus meeting standardized commercialized ideals.

In applying makeup focus less on disguising creases and more on perfecting exciting artistic looks that inspire others. Who cares about crows feet when your winged cat eye could launch trends? When conversation turns towards age, pivot to discuss adventures lived. Judge yourself and others only by growth in purposeful behaviors aligned with ethics. Stay perpetually immersed in progress and self-assurance reigns.

Exercise Authentic Self Expression

Ask trusted friends which mannerisms or Winged eyeliner style best captures personality's colorful essence. Then develop those eye expressions and cosmetic looks stopping apologetic withdrawal masking perceived imperfections. The world needs your authentic style only you can model.

Maybe slightly smudged liner and rumpled hair reflects that feisty go-getter spirit ready to rally crowds. Or dewy highlighter under gracefully hooded lids makes innocence continually reborn. However beautiful eyes manifest given genetics and era, embody it fully with chin lifted high.

Set Goals Based On Values

Rather than obsessing over static aims like perfect eyeliner wings or totally smooth undereyes, identify core values driving applause-worthy success in careers, relationships and self-mastery. What personal strengths pursued through focused goals reflect priorities and talents you uniquely offer despite aging eyes?

Get clear on contribute. Maybe you champion environmental justice issues giving a voice to marginalized communities. Or passion for Shakespeare leads to directing daring creative adaptations expanding human consciousness. Set ambitious visionary goals, get to work passionately and wrinkles become forgettable.

Control What Eye Aspects Possible

While much natural eye aging lies beyond our control without injectables or surgery, doubling down on holistic self-care legitimately within grasp makes sense. Commit to sleeping 8 hours nightly even if requires temporarily lowering social commitments.

Eat more collagen and hydration boosting foods like bone broth and cucumbers. Learn proper lymphatic drainage massage techniques for reducing puffiness. Stay committed applying premium eye creams with peptides and retinoids. Don't neglect basics that maintain function and some plumpness!

By rigorously controlling factors within your grasp like rest, diet and targeted skin care, confidence builds from restoring respectable control. And in the process eyes gleam brighter too! Cultivating confidence about our eyes amidst cultural ageism and fickle beauty constructs means rooting deeply in timeless inner wisdom that overrides fleeting appearances. Tend faithfully to self-improvement through courageous values-aligned goal pursuit. And embrace eye character lines as sacred honoring life's passionate path walked boldly. The world needs precisely what authentic eyes bravely carry.

www.ingramcontent.com/pod-product-compliance
Lightning Source LLC
Chambersburg PA
CBHW031311250726
48656CB00005B/1744